MW00624961

GROUND THERAPY

The Revolutionary Healing Paradigm
for Eliminating Pain,
Disease and Inflammation

ADELLE LABREC

Published by Think-Outside-the-Book Publishing, LLC

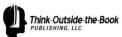

311 N. Robertson Boulevard, Suite 323
Beverly Hills, California 90211
http://www.ThinkOutsideTheBook.com

Table of Contents

Introduction

The real miracle is not to walk on water or thin air but to walk on the earth. – Thich Nhat Hanh

Imagine a healing modality so powerful that it could stop pain almost immediately—even pain that's been chronic for decades. And imagine the joyous good health you could enjoy if this same therapy could also prevent—or even reverse—a broad spectrum of serious health concerns including heart disease, disfiguring skin conditions, autoimmune disorders, cognitive and mood imbalances, and the chronic inflammation that lies at the root of virtually all modern diseases.

If all this sounds more like a utopian dream than a reality, you'll be amazed to learn about a new healing modality that can help turn your dream of vibrant, robust good health into an absolute reality.

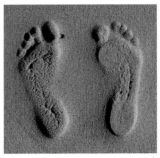

This healing modality is called "ground therapy." And it is quickly gathering momentum as a worldwide healing revolution. Ground therapy is not only incredibly effective; it is also easy to do. And because it is very inexpensive (often times, even free!) it is accessible to everyone on earth. In fact, the earth—home to all of us— lies at the very heart of ground therapy. For ground therapy starts with simply refocusing our attention on our connection with the earth.

We've all walked along the shore at the beach and felt the warm sand between our toes. Or run across a freshly mown lawn and felt the springy "aliveness" under our feet. When was the last time you stood barefoot on the earth? As a child, playing tag or chasing after fireflies? Or lying in a cool field watching the puffy white clouds paint pictures across the sky? As children, almost all of us could simply close our eyes and bring to mind the feel, the smells, and the textures of the earth. But somehow, as adults we often lose touch with these sensations. I invite you to get that feeling of freedom back. Picture yourself lying or standing in your favorite outdoor place. Imagine the feeling of soft grass under you, of warm sand trickling across your feet. If your imagination triggers memories of wonderful feelings that you experienced when you were in close proximity with the earth, you are already half way to understanding the revolutionary new healing paradigm of ground therapy.

To put it simply, we experience a very distinct kind of "feel good" when we come into direct contact with the earth. And that in itself is one good reason to spend more time outdoors. But the fact is that there's more to that special feeling than just the sense of recreation or relaxation we associate with being outdoors. In reality, the sensation we feel when we are physically in touch with the earth is a *healing* one. And this is where ground therapy truly begins—with the insight that healing occurs when our bodies and the earth touch.

Although ground therapy is still unfamiliar to most people, it is actually based on very clear, scientifically proven concepts. You see, when a direct connection occurs between our bodies and the earth, we literally soak up the earth's electrons, which triggers physical changes in our bodies. For one thing, our blood flow improves. And as we know, efficient and harmonious blood flow has been linked to overall good health and longevity. Even more impressive is the impact that ground therapy has on inflammation, which has been established as one of the most significant factors in disease onset, aging, and death. In addition, ground therapy can help prevent or reverse many other diseases and conditions that negatively impact on health, including: autoimmune disorders, cancer, fatigue, stress, insomnia, allergies, and pain (including migraines and arthritic pain).

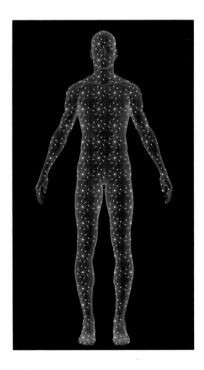

The connection between inflammation, aging, disease, and death has been documented in hundreds of breakthrough articles in publications ranging from peer-reviewed medical journals to TIME Magazine. Ground therapy's ability to quell inflammation is quite frankly an astonishing contribution to modern medicine. For this reason, many health experts are quick to say that ground therapy may be the most important health discovery of our time.

Our Disastrous Disconnect from the Earth

We invented plastics in the 1960s and immediately put those on the bottoms of our shoes. Then we carpeted our houses and built bigger and bigger houses, cutting ourselves off further from the earth. – Clint Ober, health pioneer who first discovered and documented ground therapy

The more we have tried to modernize our lives, the farther we've gotten from the earth. Our homes, cars, cityscapes, gadgets—and of course our plastic-soled shoes —all serve to "insulate" us from the natural world. But it is only relatively recently that the majority of the world's people have begun to be so radically disconnected from the earth. For most of human civilization, our forebears lived in nearly constant contact with the earth: walking barefoot on the earth's surface, sleeping on the ground, and depending on the earth for their sustenance and very survival. Their connection to the earth was primal and profound, and respect for their relationship with the earth permeated literally every aspect of their lives. The extreme importance of this connection has been recognized and revered by every ancient tradition.

In the yogic tradition, for example, feet are actually considered an extension of the *root chakra*, thought to be our body's center of survival. Our feet connect us to the earth and ground us with deep physical and spiritual security. Likewise, the ancient Ayurvedic system of health and healing in India has always acknowledged that through walking barefoot we draw energy from the earth. The concept of being "grounded" through a strong connection between our feet and the earth is similarly fundamental in other highly respected systems of healing, including yoga, Traditional Chinese Medicine (TCM), and qi gong (pronounced *chee gong*).

Perhaps it is no coincidence that all of these ancient systems are now gaining increasing attention and popularity in the West, where we are more disconnected from the earth than ever before in human history. And it is slowly becoming obvious that the price we are paying for the loss of this connection may be much costlier—and more deadly—than we've realized until now. And it is these costs that have motivated many health advocates to say that it is time to turn this trend around, to regain our connection with the earth, and to let the earth heal us through ground therapy.

Humans evolved, like all animals, walking on the ground without insulating barriers between the earth and our feet. It is common knowledge that the soles of our feet are extremely sensitive due to a high concentration of nerve endings. Since nerve tissue is electrically conductive, it is easy to understand that the bottoms of our feet are highly conductive surfaces. – Dave Gabriele, D.Ac, BA, registered acupuncturist and practitioner of Traditional Chinese Medicine

The Body Electric: The Groundbreaking Science of Ground Therapy

Ground therapy is based on the scientific principle that standing barefoot on the ground gives us access to the earth's subtle electromagnetic energies. These energies can have an enormous positive impact on our health. According to Clint Ober, the health pioneer who first discovered the benefits of ground therapy (which he calls "earthing"), when we "ground" ourselves by standing, sitting, or lying down on the earth, the earth's energies cause our bodies to become "electrically stable."

It may seem counterintuitive that our bodies are truly electrical. After all, we know that our bodies are made up of at least 60% water. Introducing an electrical charge into a body containing that much water sounds dangerous at the very least. But, scientifically speaking, the opposite is true: our bodies' systems communicate with each other constantly via *electrical impulses*. For example, the brain

6

uses electrical impulses to tell the nervous system that a stovetop is too hot. The nervous system uses the same kind of electrical impulses to tell the musculoskeletal system to move away from the hot stovetop.

Research has even demonstrated that every cell in your body may have its own natural electromagnetic field. In his book *The Body Electric*, researcher and author Robert Becker explains this intricate system of cellular communication via bioelectrical signals and natural electromagnetic fields (EMFs). These *natural* EMFs are entirely different from *man-made* EMFs, and the two types will be discussed in detail later. But in short, the critical difference between the two is that natural EMFs are actually highly beneficial to health, while man-made ones can be damaging. According to Becker, natural EMFs

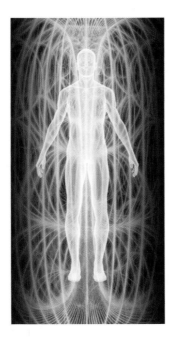

help regulate important biochemical processes of all kinds. That's why *maintaining balance* in those cellular electromagnetic fields is crucial to your physical health.

> *Human cells are not chemical in nature, but electrical. We can't expect to improve our health quickly by chemical means, because chemical reactions are relatively slow within the body. On the other hand, the effects of electromagnetism are immediate, which means that we begin to feel better right away.*

The electrical impulses within our bodies are made possible by tiny negatively charged particles called *electrons*. You may recall studying electrons in high school physics. Although electrons are far too small to be seen by even the most powerful microscope, they make up nearly all of the physical matter in our world, including our bodies and the earth itself. When we ground ourselves, we are absorbing the earth's life-sustaining electrons into our own bodies.

This process of absorbing the earth's electrons has two major positive effects on our bodies. Firstly, it helps the various systems in our bodies run more smoothly because they are able to communicate with each other without interference. And, it helps neutralize free radicals, the harmful substances that cause cell damage, accelerated aging, and chronic disease. In combination, these two effects work synergistically to prevent or reverse many of the serious ailments that afflict people living in the modern world.

Ground Therapy Provides Crucial Protection from Man-Made EMFs

Although the EMFs your body produces naturally are vital and healthy, the EMFs emitted by our man-made devices are a different and very dangerous story. As our lives grow increasingly technology-heavy and complex, we are constantly bombarded by harmful EMFs from cell phone towers, Wi-Fi routers, and other sources of electromagnetic radiation. These EMFs are making Americans sick! In fact, they are severely damaging our health without our awareness or full understanding. That's because electromagnetic radiation can penetrate our bodies, seriously compromising our health. Numerous scientists, health advocacy organizations, and environmental organizations warn that EMFs pose a disturbing array of serious health hazards. The consumer protection group SafeSpace has compiled a list detailing findings from various sources about these risks. It is, to say the least, quite shocking!

For years, scientists have conducted research linking EMF radiation to serious diseases including cancer, Alzheimer's disease, Parkinson's disease, and others. After an extensive review of 2,000+ such studies, the National Institute of Environmental Health Sciences concluded EMFs "should be regarded as possible carcinogens [cancer causing substances]." An international group of leading researchers recently stated that "the existing standards for public safety are completely inadequate to protect health."

Forward-thinking nations around the world are starting to set stricter EMF safety limits. Even the Environmental Protection Agency now cautions you to "limit your exposure."

If all these warnings from well-respected organizations, researchers, and health protection sources aren't shocking enough, mounting research suggests that EMFs may contribute to an extremely wide and varied range of health issues: brain tumors; leukemia; birth defects; miscarriages; chronic fatigue; headaches; cataracts; heart problems; stress; nausea; chest pain; compromised memory; and cancer. This list is nowhere near exhaustive, and there is strong evidence that numerous other health problems may also be linked with man-made EMFs.

Clearly, we can't eliminate all of the health-harming influences of contemporary life, such as pollution, living and working indoors, or wearing shoes. But we can take steps to minimize the negative impact of certain aspects of everyday life. And given the amount of damage EMFs can cause, and the constant onslaught of synthetic EMFs we face daily, being able to bring our bodies back into natural balance is not just one good step we can take, it's an *essential* one. Ground therapy is certainly the easiest and most reliable method of protecting ourselves from potential EMF damage, and healing from existing damage we may already have suffered—just be absorbing the earth's life-giving electrons.

The following chapters of this book will explain everything you need to know about ground therapy to achieve lasting health and wellbeing, including devices you can use to ground yourself in areas where it may not be safe to walk around barefooted. So ... are you ready to join the ground therapy revolution?

The Profound Benefits of Ground Therapy

When you ground yourself, you can expect to experience the following health benefits and more:

- Pain relief

- Instantaneously improved circulation and overall dramatic cardiovascular benefits including regulated blood pressure and more

- Anti-aging

- Dramatic increase in longevity

- Increased immunity

- Reduced stress levels and better sleep

- Drastically reduced inflammation

- Reduced risk for chronic disease

- Boosted intelligence

- Immediate improvement in skin conditions (such as psoriasis, seborrhea, acne, rosacea, etc.) because of marked change in skin conductance

- Help with healing of auto-immune diseases (lupus, Epstein-Barr, rheumatoid arthritis, multiple sclerosis, fibromyalgia, Type 1 diabetes)

- Instant allergy relief

- More strength and athletic endurance and faster recovery

- Increased energy and vitality

- Significantly reduced muscle tension

- An electron shield around your body that protects you against electromagnetic fields (EMFs) from computers, appliances, power lines, home wiring, airport and military radar, substations and transformers

Whether you go outside alone or with family, try going out barefoot: it will enhance the experience and greatly increase your overall health benefits.

Chapter One

The Ground Therapy Revolution: The Beginning

I was sitting on a park bench watching the passing parade of tourists from all over the world. At some point... my awareness zeroed in on what all these different people were wearing on their feet. I saw a lot of those running shoes with thick rubber or plastic soles. I was wearing them as well. It occurred to me rather innocently that all these people—me included—were insulated from the ground, the electrical surface charge of the earth beneath our feet. I started to think about static electricity and wondered if being insulated like that could have some effect on health. – Clint Ober, health pioneer and discoverer of ground therapy

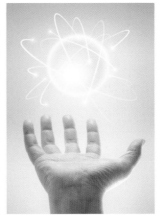

Ultimately, the most surprising thing about ground therapy is that although it is based on an extremely simple concept, it took until the 1990s for people to begin to realize its power as a healing modality. The other astounding thing is that although it is based on solid scientific principles, and has been clinically proven to be extremely effective, it has been largely ignored by the medical establishment. In fact, very few doctors are likely to even know about grounding, let alone recommend it to their patients. But that is slowly starting to change as a growing number of studies by biophysicists, medical doctors, and electro-physiologists repeatedly confirm its value as a healing tool.

Ground therapy was discovered in the 1990s by Clint Ober. At the time, Ober, a successful executive, was feeling pleased with the way his life was unfolding. He'd come a long way from his humble beginnings as a farm boy in Montana, who spend his days barefoot and out of doors, working alongside his parents and playing in the surrounding fields. Living so close to the land taught him to respect the earth not only as a source of sustenance, but also as a source of wisdom. He learned early on to "listen and learn from the ways of the natural world." Although farm life can occasionally be harsh, it can also be a very happy way for a child to grow up in balance with the earth.

Tragedy struck the family when Ober was only 15. His mother took ill, and shortly after, his father passed away from leukemia. As the eldest son, Ober had no option other than to drop out of school and tend to the farm, and to his ill mother. The years that followed were ones of hardship, but Ober credits his later success as a businessman to learning how to deal with the inevitable problems, set-backs, and difficulties of typical farm life.

In the 1960s, Ober decided to leave farm life for the excitement of the big city. He was immediately captivated by the television industry, then barely out of its infancy. The appeal of cable television for Ober was in its capacity to educate viewers and expand their horizons. "Television provided visual information to the larger world and therefore provided a window from which everyone could gain a better perspective of the real world in which they live." As we all know, television was a stellar success. And working in his chosen field, so was Ober. By the 1990s, he had built a reputation for himself as a bright and successful entrepreneur, and he had the worldly success to go along with it. Ober was enjoying the "good life;" his 5,000-square-foot mountaintop home in Colorado offered stunning views of Denver and the magnificent Rockies, and was filled with valuable art and every luxury money can buy.

But in 1993, at the relatively young age of 49, Ober found himself facing yet another potential tragedy—and this time it was his own health that was at risk. As a result of a routine root canal procedure, he developed an abscess which infected 80% of his liver, leaving it dangerously compromised. The infection swiftly spread throughout his body, causing his organs to malfunction, and putting his life in serious danger. His doctors held out very little hope that recovery was possible. On the contrary, they clearly believed that given the rapid rate at which his health was deteriorating, he had very little time left to live. Ober was advised to put his "affairs in order" and prepare himself for his imminent death.

Struggling to Live

As anyone faced with such news would be, Ober was devastated. And he was also desperate to live. So, he decided to take action on his own behalf. He consulted with a young surgeon about an experimental surgery to remove the damaged portions of Ober's infected liver. It was clear that the surgeon did not have much faith that Ober would survive the surgery, but he agreed to perform the procedure because it was Ober's only hope.

Miraculously, Ober not only made it through the procedure, but after 28 days of painful recovery in the hospital, he was released. As determined as he was to regain his health, Ober still faced a long, tediously slow, uphill battle. It took him three or four months to be able to walk a few blocks, and six months to walk a mile. But he preserved, and at nine months post-surgery, most of his liver had regenerated itself!

And then one morning Ober awoke to find that the world around him was full of a kind of beauty he'd never experienced before—"the sky a deeper blue and the trees a more vibrant green." And to his own amazement, he found that he no longer felt like a sick shadow of his former self. He felt fully, vibrantly alive! But not in the same way he'd been before his illness. His perspective had radically altered, and in a way that surprised him.

Suddenly, the stark realization hit him that he'd become a slave to his possessions, constantly striving to accumulate more material goods that would demonstrate to others his level of status and success. He says, "I never owned my home and this mountain of possessions, but rather they owned me." And with this realization, Ober decided to set himself free from his old materialistic life once and for all and dedicate himself to some more worthwhile purpose.

Although he didn't know what that worthwhile, purposeful thing would be quite yet, Ober set out to find it. He sold his house and business, bought a recreational vehicle, and hit the open road with only one goal in mind: to find his higher purpose and to discover exactly what he should be doing with his life. One night, staring across the bay at a beach in Key Largo, he idly asked himself the question that had been on his mind throughout his travels. "What *should* I be doing?" The answer was immediate— without thinking, he automatically wrote on a piece of paper, "Become an opposite charge."

Although that cryptic advice might not mean anything to most people, Ober was immediately struck by the realization that the earth's electrical impulses have life-enhancing, healing properties. He remembered how alive and healthy he'd felt as a child, running barefoot around the farm as he picked beans and milked the cows. And how ill he'd become while living in his mountaintop mansion, surrounded by beautiful scenery but entirely insulated from the earth's electrical impulses. And in that instant, the conceptual foundation of ground therapy was born.

But when Ober tried to share his discovery with others, he was almost universally met with skepticism and puzzled looks—or outright blank stares. Why would walking barefoot on the earth have any impact on the human body, positive or negative? Most people simply wrote him off, assuming that he was either a New Age mystic or a crazed quack.

A Stunning Scientific Breakthrough

Ober persevered in trying to spread his message, and as luck would have it, he eventually discovered that the National Institute of Environmental Health Sciences was compiling a paper on the effects of electromagnetic fields (EMFs) on human health. As noted earlier, EMFs are a form of radiation emitted by gadgets we use every day, such as cell phones and laptops. What Ober learned simply confirmed his suspicions; humans exposed to EMFs are prone to experiencing physiological effects, such as disturbed sleep patterns, inexplicable weight gain, and increased cortisol levels (the "stress hormone").

Interestingly, though, animals exposed to the *same* EMFs did not experience any of these adverse effects. Ober theorized that unlike humans, animals are not vulnerable to EMF damage because they are not insulated from the earth by clothing. Not only are animals naturally grounded in this way, but their bodies are also able to quickly repair and rejuvenate their cells in the absence of EMF interference.

Living in a modern world where our bodies are now constantly insulated from ground contact, we are constantly vulnerable to electrical interference from harmful EMFs. Our cells keep our bodies healthy and alive with bio-electromagnetic communications— when those communications are interrupted, disastrous consequences can and will result.

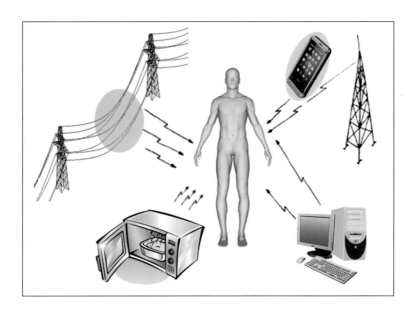

Learning about the animals' seeming immunity to the negative effects of EMFs gave Ober the inspiration for his first scientific study. The methodology Ober planned to use was elegantly simple. Participants in the study would be grounded while they slept with a grounding device, and their responses recorded. Ober chose to ground participants after they'd fallen asleep because the sleep state is when the human body undergoes most of its healing and restoration processes. In order to determine whether grounding really had the dramatic impact he anticipated, Ober's study involved dividing participants into two groups: sleepers who would be grounded, and a control group of non-grounded sleepers.

The results derived by comparing the two groups are truly astonishing. The findings Ober reported with respect to the group of grounded sleepers included the following:

- 85% of the experimental group went to sleep quicker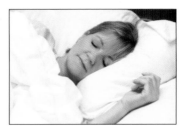

- 93% reported sleeping better throughout the night

- 100% reported feeling more rested when they awakened

- 82% experienced a significant reduction in muscle stiffness

- 74% experienced the elimination or reduction of chronic back/joint pain

- 78% reported improved general health

In addition to these very encouraging results, in later follow ups 78% of the participants in the grounded sleepers group said their general health had improved. Many also reported that sleeping grounded had also alleviated other serious health problems, including asthmatic and other respiratory conditions, rheumatoid arthritis, PMS, sleep apnea, and hypertension.

Not surprisingly, Ober was elated that this study confirmed his theory about the value of being in balance with the earth's electrical energy. But what he didn't yet know was that the benefits reported by his study subjects represented just the very small tip of a very large iceberg! In spite of the fact that there was still a lot left to learn about the benefits of grounding, Ober's results were impressive enough to encourage doctors all over the country to begin using grounding techniques with patients.

Dr. Sinatra and the
Heart Health Connection

Most notable among these pioneering physicians was Dr. Stephen Sinatra, a cardiologist at Manchester Memorial Hospital in Connecticut. Soon after starting his own medical practice, Dr. Sinatra began to notice a strange pattern emerging in his patients with arrhythmia. Their symptoms appeared to worsen around the time of each full moon. But why would his patients' health status be impacted by the phases of the moon? Granted, the moon *does* give off organic EMFs strong enough to affect the ocean tides. And the strength of the EMFs corresponds with the waxing and waning of the moon, so that at a full moon the EMFs are at their strongest.

But could that waxing and waning also affect the bodies of individual human beings? Dr. Sinatra realized that since humans are not isolated from what happens in our surroundings, and since electromagnetic events such as the waxing or waning moon can significantly impact the physical world around us, it seems highly likely that our

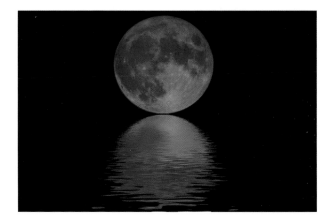

bodies could be affected by EMF events happening in the heavens as well as those happening on the earth itself.

In essence, our bodies function, for better or worse, as a collection of dynamic electrical circuits.
– Dr. Stephen Sinatra

That would explain the strange pattern occurring in Dr. Sinatra's cardiac patients on a regular, monthly basis, because the heart essentially runs on electrical impulses. In fact, it is one of the most important electrical circuits in the entire human body. Each heartbeat is triggered by an electrical signal within the heart muscle causing the heart to expand and contract, pumping blood throughout the body. When this circuit is disrupted, the heart pumps blood less efficiently, which can lead to a variety of problems including arrhythmia—and in extreme cases, heart attacks.

Dr. Sinatra wanted to explore the relationship between EMFs and heart health, so he began corresponding with Ober about ground therapy. Ober had been grounding numerous heart patients, and found that after a few short months of sleeping grounded, their health status had changed dramatically. Not only were they no longer experiencing changes in their heart conditions during a full moon, their health status was also steadily improving.

Dr. Sinatra knew that he was witnessing a radical change to the landscape of healing, a change of a much larger magnitude than he'd ever expected to see during his lifetime. Ground therapy was nothing less than revolution in full-body health, and he very much wanted to be part of that revolution.

> *With the advent of grounding, the door to a new healing frontier had been pulled open.*

But as convinced as he was about the theory behind ground therapy, Dr. Sinatra also wanted to experience it for himself. He started sleeping grounded to see what would happen, and found that both he and his wife fell asleep more quickly and stayed asleep longer. There was no doubt about it; ground therapy was a potent key for reducing stress and regulating circadian rhythms. Dr. Sinatra also suffered from psoriasis, a disfiguring and painful skin condition. But once he started reconnecting with the earth by sleeping grounded, and also by spending time fishing barefoot at a salt lake nearby, he noticed that his psoriasis improved.

If grounding could cure psoriasis, which is linked with chronic inflammation, might it also be effective for other conditions that are caused by chronic inflammation? Soon, Dr. Sinatra and Ober set their sights on a new goal— defeating chronic inflammation. Their target was not just inflammation-related skin conditions such as psoriasis, acne, and eczema, but also other serious or potentially life-threatening health problems in which chronic inflammation plays a key role.

Chronic inflammation is caused by excess free radicals in the body, and health experts across the spectrum—from researchers at the Harvard Medical School to renowned alternative practitioners like Dr. Andrew Weil—believe that it may actually be at the root of all degenerative diseases. Heart patients, for example, frequently suffer from chronic inflammation, which can lead to a hardening of the arteries, irregular heartbeat, and heart attack or stroke. When Dr. Sinatra began grounding his patients, he was delighted to see that their symptoms improved markedly.

According to the International Wellness Directory, chronic inflammation has been shown to cause the following conditions, among others:

- Depression
- Asthma
- Pancreatitis
- Parkinson's Disease
- Lupus
- Anemia
- Kidney failure
- Psoriasis
- Fibrosis
- Arthritis
- Alzheimer's disease
- Heart attack
- Stroke
- Congestive heart failure
- Cancer

The Birth of the
Ground Therapy Revolution

The health benefits of grounding were slowly but surely gaining attention in health-related circles. And the phenomenon of ground therapy really began to gain momentum with the founding of several organizations and websites devoted to researching and publicizing its potential as a healing modality, including the Earthing Institute (2010), Earthing.com and Groundology.com. As more and more people experienced the massive health benefits of grounding for themselves, they began to share their stories of healing. Clint Ober has received numerous inspiring accounts of remarkable health transformations from ground therapy users, including:

- A lupus sufferer whose joint pain decreased and mood drastically improved

- An elderly couple who experienced an ease of movement and energy level they hadn't felt in 20 years

- An allergy sufferer who found that her incapacitating reaction to pollen and cats had *completely* disappeared after sleeping grounded

- A woman who had suffered from chronic back pain for 20 years, and whose pain vanished after using a grounding mat for just *an hour and 20 minutes*

- A 14-year-old severely autistic girl whose speech and behavioral difficulties were almost completely alleviated after a month of sleeping grounded

- A 25-year-old entrepreneur who was "wasting away" from stress, and who recovered from a long and life-threatening hospital stay by sleeping grounded

- A businessman who uses grounding mats to reverse the effects of jet lag when traveling to foreign countries

- A policeman whose high-stress lifestyle and many injuries interfered with getting an uninterrupted night's sleep found that grounding allowed him not only to sleep well, but restored his energy and freedom of movement so that he was able to return to marathon running, a sport he'd been forced to give up

- An elderly medical film producer whose circulation problems had caused his feet to become blackened, cracked, and bleeding found that after five months of grounding himself, his feet returned to normal

- An acupuncturist who experienced less tension in her forearms, less professional stress, and a renewed lease on life

Enormous Benefits—Virtually Effortlessly!

The wonderful thing about ground therapy is that it offers such a vast array of health benefits, yet it is so *simple* to achieve. And it's enjoyable, too! A 20-minute barefoot walk outdoors every day is all you need. Of course not everyone has access to a place where they can walk safely outdoors. For practical reasons such as concern over toxins or pollution, or simply for lack of a space that is not completely paved over, you can also ground yourself by using a device such as a grounding mat, a special conductive sheet, or even a grounded bed. Walking barefoot on the earth is the least expensive way to ground yourself, of course, but even if you choose to use a grounding device, the cost is very inexpensive—especially when you consider the enormous benefits you'll reap.

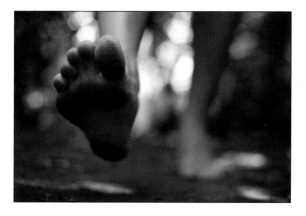

The wonderful thing about grounding is that it gives you a massive amount of benefits for a very small amount of work—less work than nearly any other alternative healing practice.

From experience, Ober developed an understanding that modern medicine is often focused on trying to obtain the greatest health rewards with the least amount of cost, whether that be measured in person hours, financial costs, resource expenditures, or a patient's pain and suffering.

The same is true about taking care of our health—and doing so in a way that isn't too "costly" in the sense of requiring drastic changes to our lifestyle. After all, our lives are busy. Abandoning our responsibilities is not an option. We cannot become nomadic hunter-gatherers or build new houses with dirt floors. We have to work around the limitations of modern life. And that is the real beauty of ground therapy; it is so easy you can quite literally do it in your sleep! Unlike many other alternative therapies that present significant financial or practical obstacles, ground therapy is available to everyone.

Chapter Two

Chronic Inflammation: The "Secret Killer"

Understanding chronic inflammation, which contributes to heart disease, Alzheimer's, and a variety of other ailments, may be a key to unlocking the mysteries of cancer. – Gary Stix

It's likely that you've heard the term "chronic inflammation" at some time or other. But most people don't fully understand what it is, or how seriously it can impact on their health. This is disturbing, because chronic inflammation is an epidemic condition of modern living, and is responsible for a wide array of health problems that attack everything from your brain to your heart to your intestines to your skin, and much, much more. For this reason, knowing how to protect yourself against chronic inflammation is crucial,

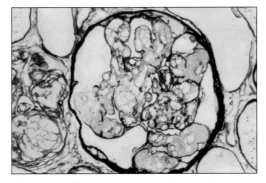

and knowing the facts will assist you in doing so. Fortunately, the seriousness of the chronic inflammation story is finally beginning to receive the media attention it deserves. For instance, a recent issue of *Time Magazine* featured a cover story entitled "The Secret Killer," which explains the link between chronic inflammation and a number of the most serious health problems we face. Another recent article in *Newsweek* called inflammation the "Alpha and Omega" of disease, and reiterated that reducing inflammation is the single most important thing we can do to improve our health and prevent disease.

> *Earthing discharges the build-up of bio-electrical stress and it supports the neutralization of free radicals that research has revealed cause pain, chronic inflammation, and auto-immune disease.*
> – Earthing USA

The Basic Facts About Chronic Inflammation

In and of itself, inflammation is not necessarily a bad thing. In fact, our bodies actually need a little bit of inflammation to survive. Acute inflammation is a healthy short-term response, mounted by our immune systems, to disruptive or potentially dangerous threats to our bodies, such as trauma, infection, and allergies. During such an episode, the immune system must distinguish between foreign, "threatening" cells and non-foreign, "non-threatening" cells. It then releases inflammatory compounds that attack the threatening cells while protecting the non-threatening ones. You can see this mechanism at work if you imagine an open cut that has become infected. The skin around it grows red and inflamed, which is a sign of acute inflammatory response that helps clear out the infected cells and protects the healthy ones from further infection. When the threat subsides (i.e. the cut is clear of infection) the swelling goes down and the cut is able to heal over. However, without this acute inflammatory response, our bodies would be unable to fight off even minor infections. That would mean that even a small nick or slight wound could potentially cause death.

Chronic inflammation, on the other hand, is a much different story. Chronic inflammation is an acute inflammatory response which *never stops*. Dr. Marcelle Pick notes that individuals whose immune system has become imbalanced tend to show *pro-inflammatory* markers even when there is no obvious infection. These markers may effectively "trick" the immune system into sensing a threat, so that it continues to release protective inflammatory compounds even in the absence of any infected cells.

At first blush this may sound like a good thing. If your body is constantly producing compounds to fight any impending threats, wouldn't that mean that you could never develop an infection in the first place? Not exactly; what actually happens is that when these floods of compounds search out infected cells to attack and don't find any, they actually being to attack and destroy *healthy* cells. Essentially, chronic infection attacks the body from the inside out.

Out of Balance

The primary cause of chronic inflammation is an imbalanced immune system. The link between the immune system, inflammation, and the development of autoimmune disorders will be fully explained later, but for now, let's take a brief look at the way our immune system functions.

Immunity involves two major systems: the *innate immune system* and the *acquired immune system.* Your *innate immune system* is in place when you are born, and it defends you from infections and illness from the minute you are born. Your *acquired immune system* is built up over a lifetime, in response to your specific daily habits, environments, lifestyle, and behaviors. These two branches of your immune system are in constant communication, trying to keep a healthy balance in your body. When this balance is not achieved, chronic inflammation is the result.

Although we have no control over our innate immune system, we *do* have significant influence over the factors that shape our acquired immunity. For example, imagine a busy ad executive living in New York City. He is constantly on his cell phone and laptop; he's on the move so much that he literally runs from meeting to meeting with little time for meals, let along healthy ones. He's likely to either skip meals, or fill up on junk food whenever he has a spare moment. His always full calendar means late nights, and his stress level allows him to catch only three or four hours of sleep a night. Although he doesn't "have time" for illness, he's plagued by various vague complaints such as headaches, stomach aches, back pain and a low level anxiety.

Someone with such a busy, stress-fueled lifestyle almost inevitably will develop immune system overdrive. His immune system will be operating on high alert, mounting constant inflammatory responses to combat the damage his lifestyle is causing: fighting minor infections with hyper force, struggling to metabolize the toxins from the junk food he consumes, and stretching itself to the limit to counteract the susceptibility to illness he has developed by inadequate sleep. This is the picture of an immune system in crisis, heading towards a major imbalance. And that imbalance opens the door wide for chronic inflammation.

How Chronic Inflammation Ruins Your Health

Medical researchers all over the world now recognize that chronic inflammation may be at the root of all degenerative disease. In part, this is because the chronically inflamed body attacks itself. The excess immune cells the body produces in an effort to stave off what it perceives as infection or threat to healthy cells begin to attack healthy muscle, ligaments, and joint fluid. The result is a sensation of pain where there should not be any, which can manifest as stiffness, general achiness, and a lack of mobility. Individuals who suffer from chronic inflammation may also develop arthritis and other forms of joint issues. And in addition, according to recent research conducted at Harvard Medical School, chronic inflammation may be linked to Type 2 diabetes and other metabolic disorders.

Severe allergic responses can also be linked to chronic inflammation, because when the immune system is constantly overtaxed while attempting to battle toxins, it can end up becoming overly-sensitive, or even entirely incapacitated. And, as Dr. Sinatra has demonstrated, chronic inflammation can play a direct role in cardiovascular disease.

Perhaps most frightening of all, it has been shown that there is a direct correlation between chronic inflammation and certain types of cancer. For instance, according to the *Journal of Clinical Investigation,* scientists at the Massachusetts Institute of Technology have found a link between chronic inflammation of the intestine or stomach and the kind of DNA damage that can result in an increased risk of developing cancer. This is because whenever our immune systems mount an acute inflammatory response to an infection, minor DNA damage is done to the inflamed cells. Normally, as soon as the immune response is over, that damage is reversed when our bodies release their anti-inflammatory compounds. But in the case of chronically inflamed cells, our bodies are unable to release these anti-inflammatory compounds and the damage to our DNA *never gets reversed* unless the underlying inflammation is treated and resolved. And cells that undergo this sort of destructive damage in this way are significantly more susceptible to cancer. [In Chapter Six, we will discuss the link between chronic inflammation and cancer in greater detail.]

Autoimmune Disorders: When Your Immune System Attacks Itself

As noted, inflammation is connected to almost every known chronic disease—from heart disease to cancer, diabetes to obesity, autism to dementia, and even depression. However, other inflammatory diseases are also rising dramatically. According to Dr. Mark Hyman, M.D., inflammation is contributing to a spike in allergies, asthma, arthritis, and autoimmune disorders. He estimates that autoimmune disease now affects a total of 24 million people.

The term "autoimmune disease" does not actually refer to one single disease. It is an umbrella term that includes a cluster of different, although related, diseases and health conditions. Rheumatoid Arthritis, Lupus, Multiple Sclerosis, Thyroid disease, Celiac disease, and Psoriasis are all considered autoimmune disorders, as are many other hard-to-classify 21st century ailments.

Dr. Hyman, a four-time *New York Times* bestselling author, is an internationally-recognized leader in the field of autoimmune issues. He is also a family physician who specializes in Functional Medicine, a ground-breaking new approach to illness. Unlike many medical perspectives that aim to treat patients' symptoms, Functional Medicine practitioners seek to identify and treat the underlying causes of chronic illness. In addition, Functional Medicine takes a "whole person" approach that views the human body as a single, integrated system, rather than as the site of various isolated symptoms. In this way, Functional Medicine practitioners are able to diagnose health issues by looking at the way various parts of the body function— and impact on each other. In other words, they are able to identify immune system dysfunctions by "joining the dots" between a cluster of symptoms that to a traditionally trained physician may seem unrelated.

Autoimmune conditions are connected by one central biochemical process: A runaway immune response also known as systemic inflammation that results in your body attacking its own tissues.
– Dr. Mark Hyman

Dr. Hyman characterizes the immune system as an "internal army" that protects you against invaders. A healthy immune system will do so by distinguishing "friend from foe." He explains that "autoimmunity occurs when your immune system gets confused and your own tissues get caught in friendly cross-fire. Your body is fighting something—an infection, a toxin, an allergen, a food or the stress response—and somehow it redirects its hostile attack on your joints, your brain, your thyroid, your gut, your skin, or sometimes your whole body."

Unfortunately, conventional drug treatments for symptoms that commonly accompany autoimmune disorders, whether they be painkillers, antihistamines, steroids, or other drugs, are often not only ineffective but also riddled with undesirable side effects. To quell systemic chronic inflammation at its source, many Functional Medicine doctors and other alternative practitioners—was well as a growing number of mainstream doctors—are now looking to ground therapy as a viable healing option.

How Chronic Inflammation
Is a "Secret Killer"

The role that chronic inflammation plays in auto-immune disorders is clear, and being diagnosed with an autoimmune condition invariably indicates the presence of inflammation. But inflammation is called the "secret killer" because it does not always manifest in this way. In fact, many people are in a state of chronic inflammation without even realizing it. While it is true that a chronic state of inflammation may produce rather dramatic and noticeable symptoms, this is not always the case. Sometimes the symptoms are relatively minor or mild, so they appear as nothing out of the ordinary. For instance, we often think of diarrhea, indigestion, weight gain, congestion, or dry eyes as simply commonplace, temporary inconveniences that everyone experiences occasionally. When we have, for instance, body aches and pains, or a skin outbreak, we rarely *view them as symptoms* at all, let alone as symptomatic of a serious health issue. Yet each of these "inconveniences" (and many more besides) can actually be warning signs that something serious is going wrong with our immune system. And unchecked, chronic inflammation in various parts of the body can lead to numerous life-threatening conditions, including:

- Atherosclerosis (inflamed blood vessel linings)

- Diabetes (inflamed pancreatic tissue)

- Arthritis (inflamed joint tissue)

- Allergies (inflamed mucosal tissue)

- Cancer (damaged DNA)

- Irritable bowel syndrome/gluten intolerance (inflamed gut tissue)

But as Dr. Marcelle Pick and other experts are quick to point out, these serious health conditions *can* be avoided. Chronic inflammation is *100% reversible*—if it is detected early and if the appropriate lifestyle changes are made. The good news is that ground therapy has been shown to be an extremely effective way to reverse the damage caused by chronic inflammation, and to prevent the onset of degenerative diseases. Ground therapy is so beneficial because it attacks the dangerous and destructive free radicals in our bodies that can damage healthy tissue. In fact, according to Earthing USA, getting grounded (or "earthing") is the *most effective* ways to neutralize free radicals.

How Does Ground Therapy Fight Chronic Inflammation?

The power of ground therapy lies in its ability to protect us from EMFs which, as mentioned earlier, promote the production of dangerous free radicals in our bodies. This is an extremely valuable attribute of ground therapy, because EMFs literally surround and bombard us all the time! Just how extensive our exposure to EMFs really is was demonstrated in a study Ober conducted. Both at home and in the workplace, the average person is constantly exposed to electrical fields that radiate from things we take for granted, such as electrical wiring and cords plugged in to wall sockets. These electrical fields alone tend to emit between 50 and 60 Hertz (Hz)—significantly more than is required to disturb the electrons in the human body, which leads to disturbances in physiological function.

> *Electric fields harm the body by disturbing and "exciting" electrons in the body, resulting in an unnatural voltage.*

This unnatural, induced voltage also encourages the production of free radicals. And as we know, the more free radicals, the more chronic inflammation. And the more chronic inflammation, the less likely the body is going to be able to produce anti-inflammatory compounds. All of this creates a vicious cycle, and our daily exposure to EMFs only adds additional fuel to the fire.

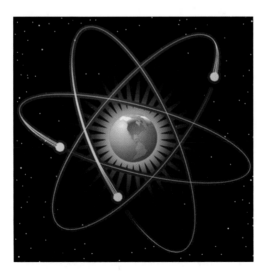

Any electrically charged object has an electrical potential, and the human body is no exception. Because our bodies—like the earth itself—experience electrochemical reactions and electrical charges, it would only make sense if they also have a voltage. And in fact, it is possible to measure the voltage of a human body with a voltmeter. When the human body is ungrounded, it will register a voltage reading that is wildly out of whack with the earth's voltage. But when grounded, the human body registers the same voltage as the earth.

What does all this talk of voltmeters and Hz mean for those who suffer from chronic inflammation? Well, the chronically inflamed body is not only unstable immune-wise—it is unstable voltage-wise too. In other words, the body's electrons are unstable, which poses a risk of structural dysfunction for an otherwise healthy cell. A cell whose electrons and voltage are out of whack will be unable to carry out its normal cellular functions, including that of ensuring that anti-inflammatory compounds are dispensed to stop an acute inflammatory response. Thus, the electrically unstable body becomes chronically inflamed.

Whereas EMFs can disrupt the natural voltage balance between our bodies and the earth, Ober's study shows that physical contact with the earth can reestablish and maintain the body's voltage in tune with that of the earth, thus ensuring that chronic inflammation cannot develop. Or to put it another way, ground therapy protects the human body from exposure to environmental toxins (including EMFs) because the earth's electromagnetic force acts as a "shield" against these harmful agents.

The Lightning Rod Analogy

If it is difficult to understand how this change in voltage could result in a change in health, use the lightning rod as an analogy. People put lightning rods on their homes in order to "ground" the lightning—that is, to send it into the ground. Imagine if your home didn't have a lightning rod and was suddenly hit by lightning: everything would be burned down. This burned down house is the equivalent of the chronically inflamed body that has gone haywire from constant exposure to all those EMFs. But what if you did install a lightning rod? The lightning would be sent into the earth, and your house wouldn't suffer the least bit of damage. This undamaged house is the equivalent of the grounded body.

Scientifically Proven Results

Ground therapy has been clinically proven to reduce chronic inflammation. In a study conducted by Dr. William Amalu of the International Academy of Clinical Thermography, 20 chronically inflamed patients who experienced grounding reported simply amazing results:

- A 65-year-old woman complaining of pain in her knees, hips, ankles, and thighs was suffering from advanced chronic inflammation that had taken away almost all her freedom of movement and left her feeling exhausted and sore. Infrared images of her hips and legs showed severe inflammation in her joints. After sleeping grounded for four nights, she reported a 91.6% reduction in pain.

- An 84-year-old woman had been suffering from an open wound on her foot for eight months; due to chronic inflammation the wound consistently failed to heal. After one week of being grounded, she experienced noticeable healing, and after two weeks the wound had healed completely. In addition, the blood circulation in her leg had improved dramatically.

- A 57-year-old man had been suffering for two years from severe foot and ankle pain caused by chronic inflammation. After sleeping grounded for only *four nights*, he reported that the pain in his feet and ankles had reduced by 80%.

- A 33-year-old female long distance runner was suffering from chronic knee pain as a result of an injury she had sustained in a race six months earlier. The pain had become severe enough to be noticeable with each step, and she could no longer run more than two miles without having to stop. After being ground for a mere half hour, she reported an immediate 30% reduction in pain. After being grounded for five days, she reported a 70% reduction in pain, and was confident she would be able to enjoy her sport again.

One of the most impressive facts about grounding is that patients reported a marked difference in their pain and swelling levels in as little as *30 minutes*. Of course, self-reports of the amount of improvement experienced can be impacted by a number of other factors, including a patient's desire to see improvement. But in this study, Dr. Amalu's methodology included infrared imaging to factually verify the level of improvement his patients experienced. And the results quite stunningly confirmed what his patients were reporting: ground therapy can not only reduce chronic inflammation, but can also do so in a matter of minutes.

The Bottom Line on Inflammation

Chronic inflammation need not be accepted as just another side effect of a modern lifestyle. Ground therapy has been clinically proven to be an extremely safe and effective means of reducing chronic inflammation, protecting our bodies from illness, and encouraging healing. In a world where we have largely become disconnected from the earth—and face the risk of serious illness because of it—don't we owe it to ourselves to reestablish our balance with the earth for the sake of our own health?

Chapter Three

Pain-Free Forever

Research has demonstrated a clearly negative influence of chronic pain on health. Now, a new study portrays a profound link between severe chronic pain and death; inflicting nearly a 70% greater mortality risk than even cardiovascular disease. – European Journal of Pain, April, 2010

The High Price of Pain

Mainstream medicine has yet to develop an effective system for managing pain. This means hundreds of millions of American must cope with pain on a daily basis. The physical, emotional, and economic costs of this pain are astronomical.

Chronic pain is epidemic; it is estimated that some form of pain currently plagues more than 100 million Americans. The most common is lower back pain. In fact, a full 80% of adults suffer—or will suffer—from lower back pain at some point in their lives, which is responsible for around 25% of all visits to primary care physicians every year. The 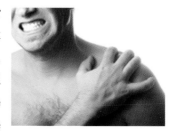 second most common is headaches, followed by joint pain (arthritic as well as trauma-related), abdominal pain, and chest pain. Aside from the physical toll that pain takes on sufferers, the financial price is also steep, both for individuals and at the national level. The top three types of pain alone—back pain, migraines, and arthritis—cost upwards of $40 billion per year. United States citizens pay approximately $600 billion annually in medical treatments and lost productivity, according to a report from the Institute of Medicine (IOM). In fact, one out of every four sick days is taken to deal with pain. And as prevalent and costly as pain is, it is poorly understood—and frequently undertreated.

What Makes Us Ache

Pain is a very individual thing, and there are also many different kinds (sharp, dull, stabbing, intermittent etc.). So, of course, there is no single cause for the pain we experience. There is, however, one common origin of the physical sensation of pain—*inflammation*. As we mentioned earlier, although inflammation is a natural part of the healing process, when it becomes chronic and ongoing, it can have a devastating impact on the body. This devastation is inextricably linked with the way that free radicals can cause cellular damage.

But contrary to common perception, free radicals are not inherently destructive. Technically, any molecule with an *unpaired electron* is a free radical. And as science reporter Natalie Angier writes in an article for *The New York Times*, "[Free radicals] are essential to many metabolic reactions in the body, they are at the heart of our immune system's ability to kill microbes, and without them we would be helpless to break down food, twitch a muscle, think a thought or reach for that bottle of vitamin supplements." One type of free radical, the *reactive oxygen species*, is generated during normal metabolic processes. Another type, *oxygen-free radicals*, is not only the most common but also the most dangerous, and can be triggered by a number of factors external to the body, such as secondhand smoke, certain foods, exercise, acute injury, or airplane travel.

It is when the body's ability to put a check on free radicals fails that damage can occur.

In other words, although we need free radicals in order to live, as Lester Packer, a biochemist at the University of California at Berkeley told Angier, they are "also the bane of our existence." Free radicals are highly reactive. It is when the body's ability to keep free radicals in check fails that the risk of damage arises. For instance, sometimes free radicals can "begin nicking [surrounding] cells to pieces," says Natalie Angier. Free radicals are normally generated as part of the body's response to trauma (such as a cut or wound) along with an influx of white blood cells. White blood cells rush to the wound site, where they perform various functions, such as killing bacteria, parasites or mold, removing debris, and initiating the healing process.

However, one crucial aspect of the white blood cell response is that as the body shifts into emergency mode to deal with the threat, it reacts with what Dr. David Gersten describes as a sort of "shotgun approach" involving the "explosive release of free radicals or 'reactive oxygen species.'" But with this "shoot first, ask questions later" approach, the wound and surrounding area is literally flooded with free radicals, often in much vaster

47

quantities than are required to quell the threat. In those cases, the excess free radicals are not expended, and enter the blood stream still "raring for a fight." It is then that they can begin to attack healthy cells and tissues, wreaking havoc on our health.

The Toll Pain Takes On Your Body

As mentioned earlier, one of the most common symptoms that arise as a result of free radicals attacking health tissue is pain. For example, arthritic pain is symptomatic of bursts of free radicals eating away at joints, stripping electrons from bones and cartilage. And when chronic pain is left untreated, under-treated, or improperly treated, numerous negative health consequences can emerge which cause additional suffering for patients. Known symptoms that can accompany—or be caused by—chronic pain include:

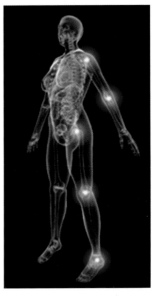

- Heightened stress

- Altered metabolic rate

- Greater risk of blood clotting

- Water retention

- Impeded healing

- Hormonal imbalances

- Suppressed immune system

- Increased risk of death

In addition, pain also takes a toll on the psychological wellbeing of sufferers, and may cause low self-esteem and feelings of worthlessness, as well as depression, hopelessness, and even suicide.

In extreme cases, long-term, treatment-resistant pain ends in suicide. One survey found that 50% of patients with chronic pain felt treatment was inadequate and considered suicide as a means of escape. Unrelieved pain also prompts requests for physician-assisted suicide, another clear sign of the severity of its impact.

How Ground Therapy Fights Pain

Ground therapy has proven outstandingly successful in relieving pain, as Dr. Gersten has observed first hand with his own patients. For example, he relates the story of Theresa, a 97-year old patient who had been battling arthritis for 15 years. Theresa's arthritis was "a relentless, progressive disease in which [she] struggled with the vicious cycle of pain, insomnia and depression," says Dr. Gersten. But after just three days of ground therapy, Theresa told Gersten that her pain had decreased by 80%.

But how—and why—does ground therapy actually *work* where so many other pain "treatments" fail? The answer lies in the way that electrons function within the body. A deficiency in electrons causes blood cells to clump together in an attempt to receive the electrical charge they are lacking. This clumping summons free radicals. But free radicals also lack electrons, which makes them interact in unstable ways, attacking healthy cells, triggering inflammation, and causing a variety of symptoms, including ongoing pain. The best way to stabilize free radicals is to correct this imbalance by supplying them with electrons. And the best way to do *that* is through ground therapy, which combats the positive charge in the body created by an excess of free radicals. Ground therapy allows electrons to flow into the body where they gravitate towards these free radicals and "partner" with them.

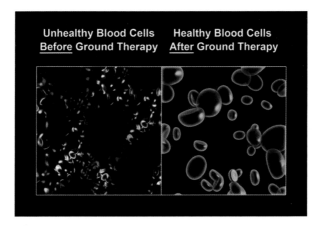

Images of human blood cells taken before and after ground therapy procedures document this phenomenon, as you can see from the image above. In the shots taken before the procedure, the blood cells are attached together in clumps. After the procedure, the cells—imbued with a negative charge from the influx of electrons—repel each other as healthy blood cells should. And as many health practitioners and patients have found, correcting this underlying electron imbalance relieves pain.

Scientifically Proven Results

The evidence concerning the effectiveness of ground therapy for relieving pain comes from many quarters, including the offices of medical practitioners, clinical studies, and scientific research initiatives. For instance, health activist Barry Davis suffered from fibromyalgia and chronic muscle tension for decades. "I have not felt good in my body for over 20 years," Davis wrote in early 2012, but after several weeks of ground therapy, he experienced enhanced physical and emotional wellbeing.

"I have had many chronic pain patients referred to me from pain management doctors," said Dr. Tracy Latz, a ground therapy expert. Many of the patients Dr. Latz sees have either had poor responses to (or are resistant to trying) medication. With ground therapy, Latz said, "they often have decreased inflammatory problems overall."

This can not only ease pain, but also address other-inflammation associated problems. "I've seen a lot of people with gluten intolerance and irritable bowel symptoms who have significantly improved by connecting to the earth," said Latz. "Their pain is better, and so is their anxiety," she says. Sometimes patients experience such profound relief that they stop grounding themselves, thinking they no longer need any pain relief. Latz then has to remind her patients that if they discontinue ground therapy, their symptoms will return.

Additional evidence for ground therapy's effects on pain comes from research conducted by Clint Ober. Subjects in Ober's study suffered from a broad spectrum of muscle and joint pains. At the conclusion of the study, every single one reported lessened pain. Each experienced positive results, including the alleviation or elimination of the following symptoms:

- Neck stiffness

- Leg and foot cramps

- Arthritis

- Carpal tunnel

- Menstrual cramps

- Headaches

- Gas and constipation

- Temporomandibular Joint disorder (TMJ)

- Joint inflammation

- Back pain

Dr. John Briffa, practicing doctor, author, and international speaker, points to a study done with 60 participants who were struggling with sleep disturbances and chronic muscle and joint pain for six months or more. Briffa divided the subjects randomly into two groups. One group slept on properly grounded mattresses while the other group used "placebo" mattresses. In other words, the participants believe that all of the mattresses had been grounded, but in fact only the mattresses used by the first group actually were.

The results were simply amazing! Of the participants who slept on grounded mattresses, 82% reported decreased muscle stiffness and pain. In contrast, *none* of the participants sleeping on the "placebo" mattresses reported any change at all in the severity of their symptoms—despite the fact that they believed they were using grounded mattresses. Biffra notes that this is not the only blind experiment to confirm the effect of ground therapy on pain symptoms; other blind experiments have also documented similar results, tracking improvement by measuring physiological responses, including heart rate, brainwave activity, and skin conductivity.

Undoing Years of Chronic Pain—Instantly!

One of the most dramatic demonstrations of the power of ground therapy occurred at the 2010 Longevity Conference. Chairman Len Foley asked the 460 attendees a simple question. "How many of you have experienced any type of physical pain anywhere in your body?" Not surprisingly, everyone in the audience raised a hand. Then Foley asked, "Is there anybody in this room who wants to get rid of your pain without doing anything—no drugs, no surgery—while you're sitting in your chair, and have the pain go away in 60 minutes?"

The room became extremely quiet. Despite the skeptical looks on many faces, Len proceeded to ask for volunteers. The criteria for volunteering were simple: participants had to have experienced acute or chronic pain for years, and they were willing to try a short procedure to evaluate whether it relieved their pain. In the end, Len recruited four volunteers, whose pain ranged from lower back pain to knee pain. Each volunteer was asked to give a small pinprick blood sample before the procedure, and another after, so that the two could be compared. The procedure itself involved affixing an adhesive patch to the bottom of each volunteer's right foot; the patch was attached to an electrically conductive grounding mechanism that had been wired to their chair.

After just one hour, the volunteers experienced freedom from the pain that they've had for years. But what was even more astounding was how their blood looked after the procedure.

The before-and-after snapshots above (page 50) are representative of the changes noticed in each volunteer's blood droplet. The "before" photo, which captured the state of the volunteers' blood cells when they were experiencing pain, shows blood cells abnormally clumped together (i.e. agglutinated). As explained earlier, this happens when the body has a deficiency of electrons and the blood cells join together in order to get the electrical charge that they need. It is this clumping effect that brings about an inflammatory response, and allows free radicals to flood the bloodstream, causing pain.

The "after" photo shows that immediately after electrons were delivered to the body via the electrically conductive grounding device, the cells detached themselves from each other. This indicates that the blood cells had become negatively charged. We know this because when healthy blood cells have their own negative electrical charge they actually repel each other, rather than clump together. This change in the state of the blood cells reflects what happened in the volunteers' bodies during grounding. Simply put, the grounding device acted as an electrical conductor, drawing electrons from the earth and delivering them to the part of the body where a deficiency in electrons existed, which was also the site of the inflammation or pain. The free radicals, which were missing an electron and so had become unstable, were immediately neutralized. And as a result the inflammation and pain completely disappeared.

A series of similarly impressive studies was carried out at an outpatient clinical treatment center in Redwood City, California. Especially noteworthy is the case of a 48-year-old woman suffering from chronic pain in both knees. The pain stemmed from a fall off a ladder six years earlier. Although she had already undergone three corrective knee surgeries, she was still unable to stand without the support of a walker. After only one 30-minute ground therapy treatment she reported a 20% reduction in pain which lasted for one full day. After five subsequent treatments, her energy increased, her pain decreased by 30%, and she felt "almost back to [her] old self." Within two weeks of beginning treatments, she felt well enough to try dancing for the first time in years, with no negative or painful symptoms afterward. After three weeks, she discarded her walker; after six weeks she was walking without even a slight limp, and after four months of ground therapy treatments, she experienced a 90% decrease in pain and swelling in both knees. Needless to say, she was beyond delighted, saying simply that "I can't believe I have my life back."

The Bottom Line on Ground Therapy and Pain

One of the most wonderful things about ground therapy is that it is so easy and inexpensive that almost everyone can do it. Although one option is to have treatments administered by a physician or other medical practitioner, another is to purchase an electrically conductive device and "ground" yourself in your own home. Considering the truly amazing capacity that grounding devices have for eliminating pain and improving well-being, you might expect such devices to sell for hundreds—or even thousands—of dollars. But actually, quality devices are extremely reasonably priced; depending on the retailer you can anticipate spending between $20 and $60 dollars.

It can be said without any equivocation that the human body evolved in contact with the earth and needs to maintain this natural contact in order to function properly. – Dr. Joseph Mercola

Dr. Joseph Mercola, a foremost voice on matters of alternative health, calls ground therapy "one of the most important overlooked factors in public health. When grounding is restored, many people report significant improvement in a wide range of ailments." Given the combination of its low cost and its impressive successes, it's easy to see why Dr. Mercola and other experts are so enthusiastic about ground therapy's potential to transform not just pain management, but the *entire practice of medicine*.

Chapter Four

Turn Back the Clock and Live Longer

But what about aging? Could chronic inflammation be the main cause of aging or a major factor accelerating aging? Can earthing slow the aging process due to its obvious and remarkable impact on inflammation?
– Gáetan Chevalier, Ph.D., Director of the Earthing Institute

The search for longevity—the proverbial "fountain of youth"—has been part of the human world since ancient times. And to some extent this quest has been 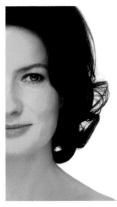 successful, when we consider that people in the developed world now have a significantly longer life span, on average, than ever before. Or to put it more exactly, the "longevity" part of the search has been successful. But simply living longer does not necessarily mean living longer in good health. And although we are living longer, the quality of life many people can look forward to in their later years may not be especially enjoyable, do to chronic illness, disease, and general poor health.

Even knowing this, for most of us the thirst to live longer remains unquenchable. Yet, the question we should be asking ourselves is whether we simply want more years, or years that are filled with health and wellbeing. When we shift our focus in this way, it is certain that the answer to this question would be that what we truly want is to live out our lives free from the debilitating symptoms of disease and disability.

However, the path to this goal has been anything but clear, because what causes aging—and its undesirable effects—has also been a puzzle to researchers. But that is beginning to change, as more researchers and health professionals discover proof that inflammation is one factor that plays a seriously destructive role in the aging process. Alongside this knowledge, it is becoming increasingly clear that health decline is not an inevitable consequence of aging. And because of ground therapy's incredible ability to reduce the chronic inflammation that leads to a decline in general health, as well as to serious diseases, it has an extremely valuable role to play in helping protect our health as we grow older.

How Aging Ravages Our Bodies

Age may be "just a number," as many people say, but the process of aging is not purely the result of the accumulation of years. There are many factors involved in aging, and improving the health of people as they age can help stave off many of the more devastating effects of the encroaching years. As Gáetan Chevalier says, one of the most important goals of modern medicine should be focused on improving the health of older people.

Dr. Chevalier, the director of the Earthing Institute, is a visiting researcher at the Developmental and Cell Biology Department, University of California at Irvine. He is also a highly regarded scientist, and his experiments looking at the bioelectrical changes brought about by grounding have opened a new frontier of electrophysiological research. Dr. Chevalier was also formerly the director of research at the California Institute for Human Science in Encinitas, California, a leading center for the investigation of healing applications of subtle energies.

> *It is imperative to decrease the alarming rate of hospitalization, risky and frequently injurious administration of multiple medications, and soaring age-related disease-care costs.*
> – Dr. Gáetan Chevalier

So, what exactly does the process of aging involve? And how does this process impact on our health? As we age, the productivity rate of our tissues and cells slows down. Consequently, the body's capacity to absorb and metabolize nutrients declines. This process is "further compromised by drug side effects and interference," notes Dr. Chevalier. Though at least 300 separate theories have been proposed to explain the physiological degradation that accompanies *senescence* (aging), none has thoroughly mapped the impact of aging on the body's *immunobiology* (functioning of the immune system). As the body ages, so does the immune system. One characteristic that is typical in this immune system aging, or *immunosenescence*, is the presence of chronic low-grade inflammation. In fact, inflammation is so commonly linked to aging that some researchers have dubbed it "inflamm-*aging*."

Recent, provocative scientific findings indicate that the physical changes we associate with aging are actually side effects of inflammation.

The body's inflammatory system is an essential defense against diseases. However, a lengthy history of battling contagions leaves severe collateral damage, including the effects discussed in Chapter Two. And as Russell Tracy, professor of pathology and biochemistry at the University Of Vermont College Of Medicine, notes, "Inflammatory factors predict virtually all bad outcomes in humans."

Inflammation Drives the Aging Process

Much like the classic question of whether the chicken or the egg came first, scientists have yet to fully comprehend the complex connection between aging and inflammation. We do know that from an evolutionary perspective, strong immune and inflammatory responses were necessary to allow humans to survive to reproductive age. Of course, until quite recently lifespans were relatively short; as lifespans have lengthened considerably, researchers are finding that over time, the cumulative impact of these same responses can lead to very detrimental consequences. For instance, molecular and cellular damage caused by inflammation can lead to loss of organ functionality, the collapse of structural integrity, greater susceptibility to diseases, and an increased likelihood of death.

One of the dominant theories concerning the interplay between aging and inflammation focuses on the role of free radicals. As discussed earlier, free radicals cause damage when too few electrons are present within the body to counteract them. With respect to aging, the theory suggests that the physical deterioration that accompanies aging is also caused by free radicals. Free radicals impact the body in three critical ways that may cause the specific type of damage typically seen in age-related bodily breakdown: DNA damage and mutation; deterioration or self-destruction of the mitochondria; and protein cross-linking (proteins sticking to each other). With respect to protein cross-linking, in which free radical damage causes proteins to clump together, the efficiency of enzymes is reduced, which would explain certain visible signs of aging, such as skin wrinkles. As Dr. Nicholas Perricone, bestselling author of *7 Secrets to Beauty, Health, and Longevity* puts it, "Aging skin is [skin that is] inflamed on the inside."

Under Fire! Inflamm-Aging

Over the last decade or so, chronic inflammation—and its links with disease—have received quite a bit of attention in the media, as well as in academic publications. But the truth is that this link does not represent a "new" discovery. In fact, medical experts have been probing the connection since the 19th century. These investigations received a huge boost with the emergence of modern biochemistry, which allows scientists to parse the intricate chemical pathways of the body's inflammatory response. With this deeper understanding, we now know that although the body's inflammatory defense mechanism is absolutely essential to life, when it is overwhelmed so that it cannot shut itself off, it can do more harm than good. In essence, chronic inflammation ensues, which results in poisoned organs and damaged tissues. And as mentioned earlier, inflammation now appears to be the source of all the chronic conditions, including those most commonly associated with aging, such as diabetes, atherosclerosis, Alzheimer's disease, and heart disease.

These inflammation-related chronic diseases represent leading causes of death for aging adults. In fact, older adults are disproportionately at risk for disease and injury: roughly 80% have one chronic disease, and 50% have two or more. That is why the Centers for Disease Control and Prevention noted in a 2011 report that "an essential component to keeping older adults healthy is preventing chronic diseases and reducing associated complications." Given the clear and direct link between inflammation and chronic disease, it is not difficult to see why reversing inflammation is the single most important factor in protecting health as we age.

How Ground Therapy Stops the Clock

As we all know, antioxidants are the natural enemies of free radicals. But what you may not know is that the free electrons that ground therapy transfers from the earth into the body are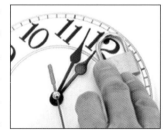

actually antioxidants, and in fact they are among the most *potent antioxidants* available.

Dr. James Oschman, who holds degrees in biophysics and biology and is an expert in the field of energy medicine, says that the body appears to be "designed with a semi-conductive fabric that connects everything in the body." This "living matrix," as Oschman calls it, is composed of a gel-like material called *ground substance*. This gel stores electrons, so in effect, "the whole fabric is basically an antioxidant defense system that is in every part of our body," explains Oschman. Ground therapy supports this system by flooding your body with an abundance of electrons, encouraging it to return to its optimal electrical state. When your body is electrically balanced, it is able to function more efficiently with respect to self-regulation and self-healing, as well as in reducing inflammation.

According to Dr. Mercola and other experts, free electron antioxidants are your best defense against free radical damage. Once the free electrons enter your body, seeking out and neutralizing free radicals, significant clinical changes occur in factors related to premature aging, including decreased levels of inflammation, beneficial changes to heart rate, and a decrease in skin resistance.

Scientifically Proven Results

"Can [ground therapy] reduce the severity and incidence of chronic illness and extend the quality and quantity of life? We seriously think so," says Dr. Chevalier.

"It is not a panacea," Chevalier says, "but it sure may be a difference in how long and well we live." Since the publication of Clint Ober's pioneering book, health professionals worldwide, including Dr. Chevalier, have documented major health improvements in thousands of cases. Based on evidence from thermography images, Dr. William Amalu, president of the International Academy of Clinical Thermography, agrees that ground therapy "significantly reduces inflammation." Thermography is not only able to identify areas of inflammation, but can also show the level of severity. Typography scans produce color-coded "maps" which reflect the relative temperature in various spots on the body. The hotter the area, the more yellow, orange, and red will appear on the scan. And because the greater the inflammation in the affected area, the hotter it will be, the degree and severity of the inflammation can both be determined from the same scan.

Based on clinical observation and double-blind research studies, [ground therapy] is now fully integrated into my practice of nutritional medicine. The power and simplicity . . . cannot be over-estimated. It is an infinite supply of free electrons, which enter our bodies and neutralize the free radicals that cause inflammation.

— Dr. David Gersten, in Vision Magazine

Scans done pre- and post-ground therapy interventions show normal thermal symmetry in the latter scans, indicating decreases in inflammation. Oschman describes ground therapy as turning on "an anti-inflammatory switch" which helps our bodies to normalize, so that damage is reduced and aging prevented.

The Bottom Line on Ground Therapy and Anti-Aging

According to experts, a 30-minute barefoot walk each day will accelerate the anti-aging and anti-inflammatory effects of ground therapy. Statistics indicate that roughly 30 million people in the United States intentionally find time to "go barefoot" for this very reason. Of course, the more time you spend grounded, the more plentiful the benefits, and the faster they appear. Clearly, it is not practical for most of us to spend countless hours walking barefoot outdoors, but grounding devices can also provide you with a steady source of free electrons which will also amplify the benefits to your body.

"As someone who has participated in numerous earthing studies," says Chevalier, "it is obvious to me that routine contact with the earth offers a powerful intervention against chronic illnesses by decreasing or eliminating inflammation." In conjunction with the other benefits of ground therapy, this leads to increased stress resistance. "By reducing stress, earthing improves the ability of the body to survive," explains Chevalier. What could be a more potent anti-aging aid than that?

Chapter Five

Stop Stress—the "Stealthy Attacker"

Stress-related diseases are an important cause of death for many animals, including humans. In addition to the harmful effects of the factors causing the stress in the first place, responses to stress often have their own detrimental effects. – Dr. Lilach Hedany, *Proceedings of The Royal Society of Biological Sciences*

The connection between stress and health issues, including disease and death, is now well established. Dr. Stephen Sinatra has studied the effects of ground therapy 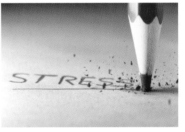 on human stress levels and has found it to be incredibly beneficial for calming down the stress response. According to Sinatra and other experts, grounding has been shown to dramatically reduce stress levels and heal the damage done to the body by stress.

But just how does ground therapy work to get rid of stress?

According to experts, grounding the body calms the nervous system, reducing the negative effects of our "fight-or-flight" stress response. It also helps reduce chronic stress by removing stress-inducing compounds such as cortisol and adrenaline from our bloodstreams. This is the "in a nutshell" explanation, but to truly understand how ground therapy works on stress, we need to take a step back and look at what stress is, what causes it, and how it can harm our health.

By encouraging activity in the parasympathetic branch [of the nervous system], grounding helps people relax and reduce stress. – Dr. Stephen Sinatra

It's Never "Just" Stress

"Stress"—everyone's least favorite six-letter word—and, apparently, something that the majority of us worry about. In fact, according to a recent study by the American Psychological Association, more than half of all working adults (and a full 47% of *all Americans*, working or not) say that they are very "concerned with the amount of stress in their lives." A heightened awareness of stress as a health issue, and perceptions of the role stress plays in daily life may, of course, underlie part of this concern. But the actual level of stress that we experience on a day-to-day basis also appears to be escalating, as compared to only a few decades ago.

For instance, a research study conducted at Carnegie Mellon University in Pittsburgh has revealed that stress levels (as measured by accepted tests) for both men and women have increased by at least 20% since 1983. If stress levels can rise so quickly in the space of a short 30-year span, just imagine how much more stress we face than our ancestors of 100 years ago. The same study found, moreover, that stressed-out Americans are more likely to be suffering from hypertension, anxiety, depression, and obesity. This correlation suggests that the more stressed out we get, the more negative health habits we acquire in order to cope with our stress. This is a vicious cycle, because as those negative habits take their toll on our health, we find ourselves burdened by even more stress in the form of illness.

But the cycle is actually even more complex and vicious than that, because stress makes you more susceptible to illnesses. According to a review in the *Observer* (December 2007), the magazine of the Association for Psychological Science, stress plays an instrumental role in lowering our resistance to everything from the common cold to erectile dysfunction and gum disease. Research shows that chronic stress has also been linked to heart disease, intestinal problems, growth problems, Type 2 diabetes, skin disorders such as psoriasis and eczema, depression, and posttraumatic stress disorder. In addition, the excessive levels of stress hormones that are released into the body by chronic stress have been shown to accelerate the growth of precancerous cells and tumors; they also lower the body's resistance to HIV and cancer-causing viruses like human papilloma virus (the precursor to cervical cancer in women).

In other words, as scientists have long suspected and now are able to confirm, stress actually *does* kill. And it does so in stealthy, widely varied ways. When we live with constant high stress, we are putting our very lives at risk.

Making an effort to reduce stress in our lives is clearly well worth it.

In order to understand how reversing the negative effects of stress with ground therapy translates into enormous positive health benefits, it is helpful to understand the science of stress.

What Fuels Stress in the Body?

As a physiological phenomenon, stress has existed since time immemorial. In fact, it is a crucial component of our evolutionary success. Both cave-dwelling humans and primates depended upon the stress response for survival.

Stanford neuroendocrinologist Robert Sapolsky, who studies the stress response in humans and primates, explains why stress was once the body's surefire mechanism for avoiding danger. When primates perceive a threat, their endocrine systems kick into high gear, releasing a series of hormones—especially epinephrine (cortisol), norepinephrine, and adrenaline—from the adrenal glands above each kidney. These hormones increase the primate's heart rate, boost respiration, and increase the availability of glucose in the animal's blood. Glucose is the body's cellular fuel; we metabolize it in order to carry out all of our daily activities. The increase in glucose during the "fight or flight" response gives the animal a boost of energy; coupled with the release of hormones that sharpen his mental acuity, this energy boost allows him to deal with the threat, either by confronting the danger or fleeing to safety.

Because the stress response takes so much energy, the body often has to adjust accordingly. Survival is the priority in the face of danger; thus speed and strength are critical, and the systems that oversee those functions go into overdrive. But other functions, such as those performed by the digestive, reproductive, and immune systems fall quite low on the priority scale until the danger has passed, so these functions slow down considerably. For our early ancestors, dangers usually passed quite quickly, and the body was able to dial down the stress response after five or 10 minutes in the heightened state and return to normal functioning.

Unfortunately, the same is not true for present-day humans. Although we rarely encounter life-threatening stressors in our daily lives, work in relatively safe environments and return at the end of the day to even safer homes, we are more stressed than our ancestors! In fact, many of us are in a chronic state of stress. Instead of having our fight or flight response activated for very brief periods of time to face real dangers, many of us have permanently "turned on" stress responses that are due to purely *psychological* reasons. Perhaps we are worried about an impending meeting with a boss, a child who is underperforming at school, or missing the bus to work and being late—again. Whatever the immediate worry, our bodies are in a heightened state of tension until the problem is resolved. And when we have many of these kinds of worries on our minds, our bodies are continually being flooded with the "fight or flight hormones." But rather than dissipate, these hormones remain in our systems for months at a time. The human body was clearly not designed to withstand long periods of sustained stress, so is it any wonder that keeping it in a chronic state of "high alert" can cause serious health problems to develop?

If you turn on the stress response chronically for purely psychological reasons, you increase your risk of adult onset diabetes and high blood pressure. If you're chronically shutting down the digestive system, there's a bunch of gastrointestinal disorders you're more at risk for as well. – Robert Sapolsky

How Stress Makes You Old and Sick

One of the detrimental side effects of chronic stress, according to beauty and skincare researcher Danna Norek, is damage to our DNA, which causes us to age more quickly and ultimately reduces our lifespans.

Stress causes destruction to our telomeres, which are protective proteins that bind strands of DNA together. Damaged *telomeres* can cause DNA to give cells erroneous information about how to behave. Healthy DNA may instruct cells to make more protein, for instance, to 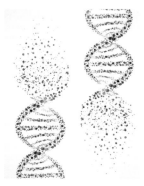 keep our skin, hair, and teeth stronger. Damaged DNA, on the other hand, may either fail to transmit these messages, or may send the wrong—and sometimes deadly

—instructions to our cells. Telomere damage can lead to a number of stress-related illnesses like diabetes, heart attacks, and even cancer. In fact, the list of ailments caused by stress is staggeringly long, and there is clearly no longer any question that the impact of chronic stress on our lives is largely negative. And although we've mentioned quite a few, there are other health issues that may not be so obviously linked with stress, such as the ones below.

Insomnia: Stress interferes with our ability to sleep. Because much of the repair and rejuvenation of the body occurs while we are asleep, a sleep-deprived body is more prone to illness, chronic infection, and psychological disorders than a well-rested body.

Poor Eating: Eating junk food is an incredibly common method of coping with stress. Long-term over-consumption of sugar, unhealthy fats, salt, and food additives causes serious problems. Poor eating is the number one reason that stress has been linked to degenerative conditions like Type 2 diabetes and obesity.

Depression: Stress and depression are closely linked. Long-term depression can negatively impact your life in a number of ways, causing you to become more distant from your friends and loves ones, lose your enthusiasm for activities your normally enjoyed, and slow your metabolic rate. In extreme cases, depression can lead to suicide.

Circulatory Problems: During the fight or flight response, hormones constrict your arteries in order to prepare you to perform a series of strenuous tasks in a short period of time. But when those arteries stay constricted for a long period, they can reduce blood flow throughout the body and create major problems such as blood clots and poor circulation. In extreme cases, they can even lead to strokes.

Sexual Dysfunction: The stressed-out body shuts down a number of its systems, including the reproductive system. If your body is in a chronic state of stress, you can expect to experience a radically diminished sex drive. Men may experience erectile dysfunction and premature ejaculation.

Growth Problems and Accelerated Aging: According to Sapolsky, children under stress can experience a syndrome called Stress Dwarfism, which seriously stunts their growth. This is because the chronically stressed body is unable to produce as much Human Growth Hormone (HGH) as it normally would. In bodies that are already fully grown, a lack of HGH can interfere with cellular repair and lead to aging and disease.

Prolonged Systemic and Local Infections: The stressed out body has a weaker immune system, which means it has a harder time fighting off a common cold, healing an infected wound, and combating viruses like HIV and the cancer-causing human papilloma virus (HPV).

Cancer: A chronically stressed system has both damaged DNA and the inability to correct for damages in that DNA. To make matters worse, it has been shown that chronically elevated stress

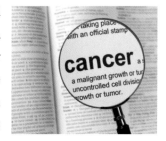

hormones have been known to accelerate the growth of precancerous cells and cancerous tumors, which means that the likelihood of developing full-blown cancer is significantly increased.

Of course, knowing that you are in a chronically stressed state should encourage you to make the necessary changes in your life to reduce stress. But stress can be a difficult thing to recognize, especially when we are accustomed to the demands of a fast-paced, high-stress world. We may become so used to thinking of stress as just part and parcel of being alive that we don't even really realize that we have become over-stressed. The symptoms listed below may help you determine whether you are chronically stressed, or if the stressors in your life are putting you at risk of becoming so.

- Sleeplessness or sleep disturbance
- Gastrointestinal dysfunction (indigestion, heartburn)
- Weight gain
- Anxiety or paranoia
- Frequent susceptibility to colds and viruses
- Cuts or wounds that do not heal
- Stiffness in your joints
- Muscular aches and pains
- Difficulty waking up or staying awake
- Frequent, insatiable hunger

Even if you have none of these symptoms, making efforts to reduce stress will help you avoid these—or more serious—health issues in future. But you may wonder how it is possible to reduce stress without radically changing and simplifying your life. If so, you'll be happy to hear that such drastic measures are usually not necessary. Ground therapy can help you reverse chronic stress easily and quickly.

Although chronic stress is dangerous to our health, the effects of stress are 100% reversible. Ground therapy can equip us with the tools we need to recover our bodies and restore our minds from a state of chronic, degenerative stress.

How Ground Therapy Quells Stress

When we are not grounded, our voltage is out of whack with the earth's voltage and we are vulnerable to the numerous EMFs in our daily environments. This causes our bodies' electrons to be in an excited state. This "excited state" means that our bodies have a harder time performing functions that are normally routine: it is harder for cellular messages to be relayed; harder for the body's systems to communicate and synchronize; and harder for crucial repairs to take place.

A body bombarded by EMFs is going to find itself in a state of chronic stress, which means that it will overproduce hormones such as cortisol. As mentioned earlier, cortisol is one of the key hormones produced during the fight or flight response. And while it is extremely valuable in such instances, too much cortisol in the blood can be harmful, leading to sleep disturbances, obesity, and depression, among other negative health effects. Ground therapy lowers our cortisol levels to a normal, healthy range.

It does so by grounding our bodies. A grounded body is not so vulnerable to EMFs in its environment. Its electrons return to a normal, non-excited state and the body's cellular and systemic functions are not charged with the difficult tasks of communicating with each other through the interference of harmful EMF radiation. Because a grounded body is less stressed, it produces less cortisol. This means that it is easier for the grounded individual to fall asleep and stay asleep, as well as recover from long-term injuries and stave off infections.

Medical researchers have found that after just a few nights of sleeping grounded, chronically stressed patients have shown the following improvements:

- An easier time falling and staying asleep

- Reduced stress-related anxiety

- Reduced pain

- An easier time battling infections

- Weight loss

- Looking/feeling much younger

Scientifically Proven Results

· Ground therapy has marked benefits for the chronically stressed body, many of which have been scientifically shown to *permanently reverse* the negative effects of chronic stress. Of special significance is the fact that grounding has been demonstrated to normalize cortisol levels. For instance, a study by Dr. Maurice Ghaly and Dr. Dale Teplitz provides concrete evidence of improved cortisol levels with subjects who slept grounded. Their findings were published in the *Journal of Alternative and Complementary Medicine* (2004). In their article, entitled "The Biological Effects of Grounding on the Human Body During Sleep as Measured by Cortisol Levels and Subjective Reporting of Sleep, Pain, and Stress," the authors detailed both their methodology and findings.

A total of 12 subjects were chosen for the study, each of whom reported experiencing sleep dysfunction, pain, and stress. Prior to the start of the study, both the subjects' voltage and circadian cortisol levels were measured. These measurements allowed the researchers to identify irregularities in the participants' test results as compared against normal levels. A balanced voltage reading would fall somewhere around the same voltage as that of the earth, which is typically far below 1.00. However, at the onset of the study, all subjects clearly had an electrical imbalance, with readings above 1.00.

The circadian cortisol test, which maps fluctuations in cortisol levels throughout the day, showed that all 12 subjects had an irregular, disturbed pattern of cortisol production, as well. In a healthy person, cortisol is produced in a pattern that is conducive to the normal sleep-wake cycle. Cortisol levels will typically be highest in the morning, which coincides with waking up, and then slowly decline throughout the day until around 9 pm, which makes us feel prone to sleepiness and allows us to fall asleep.

This is not the case in the chronically stressed body, however. Because the fight or flight mechanism is permanently stuck at "on" the body is constantly working overtime, which means that it's constantly producing cortisol. In the pre-trial testing, subjects were producing cortisol at all hours of the night, which is the reason they were experiencing insomnia.

In preparation for the study, each participant was provided with a grounding mattress pad, and was asked to fill out daily sleep diaries and weekly pain surveys to record how they felt during the course of the 8-week study. After a mere eight weeks, all 12 subjects reported that their various ailments, such as sleep dysfunction, pain, and stress, were either greatly reduced or *eliminated altogether*. Based on their self-evaluation of their symptoms, the following results were obtained:

- All 12 subjects reported waking fewer times during the night

- Nine of the 12 subjects reported experiencing less fatigue in the morning

- Ten of the 12 subjects reported decreased pain

- Seven of the 12 subjects reported that their pain no longer interfered with their daily activities

- Nine of the 12 subjects reported an improvement in their daytime energy levels

- Nine of the 12 subjects reported a dramatic reduction in their emotional stress levels

The clinical measurements taken after the study provided objective support for the improvements participants reported. The subjects' voltage levels had all dropped to below 1.00. In addition, their cortisol production has begun to normalize, with cortisol production occurring only during the day and following the circadian pattern typical of individuals in good health.

These dramatic results confirmed the value of ground therapy in dealing with sleep disorders, pain, and stress. But a number of other unexpected benefits also came to light through this study. For instance, six of the seven subjects who reported gastrointestinal disorders prior to sleeping grounded reported improvement.

Of the six female subjects who reported problems related to PMS or hot flashes before being grounded, five subjects reported a dramatic decrease in symptoms. And all three subjects who reported experiencing TMJ and other joint pain prior to sleeping grounded reported a decrease in symptoms after the eight-week experimental period.

The Bottom Line on
Ground Therapy and Stress

Chronic stress is not simply an inconvenience, it is dangerous; in fact, it is one of the silent killers of modern society. Although we live with chronic stress every day, and many of us have become experts at ignoring it, we do so at our own peril. Living longer and healthier lives means paying attention to the stress cues in our lives, and taking steps to reduce or eliminate the risks associated with chronic stress wherever we can. Often the health advice we receive from experts, doctors, and others may seem complicated and unrealistically difficult—a case of the "cure being worse than the illness." But in this case, nothing could be further from the truth! Becoming more grounded and balanced is as simple as spending a few minutes a day walking barefoot, or sleeping with a grounding mat. After all, we have enough stresses in our lives; taking steps to de-stress shouldn't be the source of yet another stress.

Chapter Six

Turn Off the Fuel that Feeds Cancer

The link between inflammation and cancers, rather than a recent concern, was noticed 150 years ago. As early as 1863, Virchow indicated that cancers tended to occur at sites of chronic inflammation. – Dr. Haitan Lu, in the journal *Molecular Cancer Research*

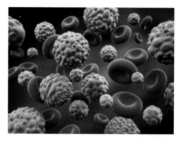

The link between cancer and ground therapy is a simple equation: when we are disconnected from the earth we are at risk for developing cancer; when we restore our balance with the earth we can reverse those risks. How? Well, in a nutshell, one of the factors directly linked with cancer is the oxidative stress load in the human body. Ground therapy reduces oxidative stress, which effectively neutralizes that cancer risk.

Research shows that ground therapy during sleep is an excellent, effortless way to reduce oxidative stress and inflammation in your body.

Of course, the details of how ground therapy works to prevent cancer is slightly more complicated than that. To fully appreciate the beauty of what ground therapy can do in this respect, it helps to have a more in-depth understanding of cancer itself, and of why it is often described as the most dreaded disease that exists.

Cancer: The Most Dreaded of All Diseases

Almost no one can hear the word "cancer" and not feel that pinch of dread in the stomach. There's good reason for that. Cancer is one of the deadliest diseases known to humankind. According to research conducted by the World Health Organization, 12.6 million people around the world are diagnosed with cancer every year, and more than 7.5 million die of the disease. That means that virtually every one of us is familiar with the devastation cancer can cause, either personally or by knowing someone who has faced the "voracious beast" that is cancer. The National Cancer Institute recently compiled a list of the most common types of cancer along with the predicted cases for 2013 and the number of deaths for each (see chart on next page).

The sheer immensity of suffering that these numbers represent is alarming. And more alarming still, these numbers are steadily increasing. The American Cancer Society's prediction for 2012 was that roughly 1,638,910 new cases of cancer would be diagnosed, and of these, approximately 577,190 would prove to be fatal. This equates to more than 1,500 cancer deaths *per day*! Cancer is considered to belong to the category of illnesses described by the World Health Organization as *lifestyle* diseases, which also includes such conditions as diabetes, hypertension, obesity, heart failure, and stroke. Lifestyle diseases are *non-communicable* (non-infectious, nontransferrable) diseases, which means that they cannot be passed from one person to another but originate from factors inherent in an individual's lifestyle, broadly construed to include such factors as genetic background, environment, exposure to toxins, as well as lifestyle habits such as diet, exercise, smoking, alcohol use etc.

Type of Cancer	Predicted Cases	Predicted Deaths
Bladder	72,570	15,210
Breast	232,340 (female); 2,240 (male)	39,620 (female); 410 (male)
Colon and rectal	102,480 (colon); 40,340 (rectal)	50,830 (combined)
Leukemia	48,610	23,720
Lung	228,190	159,480
Melanoma	76,690	9,480
Pancreatic cancer	45,220	38,460
Prostate	238,590	29,720
Non-Hodgkin Lymphoma	69,740	19,020
Thyroid	60,220	1,850

Granted, we have control over many of these factors, but of course, not all. But it is clear that the threat of developing cancer is a very real one, and we owe it to ourselves to take every possible preventative measure we can to protect ourselves. The old advice to "know thine enemy" is especially pertinent here, because the more we understand about cancer, its causes, and its symptoms, the better armed we will be to fight against it.

What Fuels Cancer?

There are many potential answers to this question, ranging from theories about the molecular makeup of the human body to a laundry list of bad lifestyle habits that must be avoided. According to the UK Cancer Research Institute, the causes of cancer can be divided up into roughly eight categories: carcinogenic (cancer-causing) substances; age; genetic makeup; immune system imbalances; lifestyle choices; daily environment; viruses; and bacterial infections.

Carcinogens

Carcinogenic substances are cancer-causing toxins such as those found in cigarette smoke, many chemicals, and various food additives, to name just a few.

Age

While DNA changes that ultimately result in a cell becoming cancerous can begin at any time, the process often takes many years. This means that the more years that we accumulate, the more time these cells have to develop into cancer somewhere in the body.

Genetic Makeup

Some people are born with a genetic mutation at the cellular level which can ultimately cause the cells to become cancerous. While individuals who have a particular genetic mutation are more predisposed to developing cancer, the presence of such a genetic mutation does *not* mean that cancer is inevitable. A number of other factors may also be involved, and although scientific research into the links between these factors is still inconclusive, research is ongoing.

The Immune System

A healthy immune system is critical for fighting cancer, because when the immune system is functioning well, it has the ability to recognize, attack, and eliminate mutated cells. On the other hand, a compromised immune system may be incapable of fighting off threats to cells, which leaves individuals with weak immune systems more prone to developing cancer.

Lifestyle Choices

Almost everyone is aware that smoking is directly linked to cancer. But many people do not know that other factors related to lifestyle, such as excess weight, too little physical activity, and poor diet also increase the risk of cancer. For instance, the standard diet of many Americans, which relies heavily on red meat and processed foods, does not provide enough of the nutrients (such as those found in fruits and vegetables) to keep our immune systems healthy.

Environmental Factors

Environmental factors that can lead to cancer include— but are not limited to—secondhand tobacco smoke, excessive exposure to the sun, workplace hazards (such as EMFs from workplace technologies), asbestos, and both natural and man-made radiation.

Viruses

Viruses, which disrupt, destroy, or compromise the genetic structure of healthy cells, can encourage the onset of cancer-causing processes.

Bacteria

Recent research has shown that bacterial infections may be linked to certain stomach and digestive tract cancers. Humans with a helicobacter pylori (H pylori) infection of the stomach have developed inflammation in the stomach lining, which increases the risk of developing cancer.

The Cruel Cost of Cancer

Cancer need not be a death sentence—if it is caught early, cancer can be cured. But in order to catch it in time, we need to know what symptoms to be on the lookout for. According to the American Cancer Society, symptoms that are cause for concern and that warrant a visit to your physician include:

- Unexplained weight loss

- Persistent fever

- Fatigue

- Chronic pain

- Changes in coloration of the skin

- Change in bowel habits or bladder function

- Sores that do not heal

- White patches in the mouth or white spots on the tongue

- Unusual bleeding or discharge

- A thickening or lump in the breast or other soft tissues

- Indigestion or trouble swallowing

- Recent growth or change in the texture or shape of a skin wart or mole

- Nagging cough or hoarseness

Recognizing these symptoms early on is crucial for our health and survival, and we urge all readers who experience any of these symptoms to report to their family doctor or health care professional as soon as possible. And given the drastic costs of cancer, both in terms of suffering and loss of life, we urge everyone interested in protecting themselves from this devastating disease to consider what ground therapy has to offer in this respect.

Cancer Protection With Ground Therapy

As mentioned briefly earlier, one of the most significant contributing factors to lifestyle illnesses such as cancer is *oxidative stress. Oxidation* is the process by which our cells produce energy by taking in oxygen and pushing out carbon dioxide, and occurs within our bodies hundreds of millions of time a day. In the process of oxidation free radicals are often produced. And while these are free radicals of the harmful variety, in a healthy person with normal oxidation levels they are typically cleared up quite rapidly by the body's natural antioxidants.

But a major problem arises when the body is over-taxed, and free radicals are being produced at too fast a rate for the antioxidants to clear them away. This creates a state of oxidative stress within the body, which can lead to a number of negative implications, including structural damage to cells, reduction in cellular activity, and dysfunctional cellular activity. Oxidative stress has been linked to diseases as diverse as asthma, carpal tunnel syndrome, diabetes, and cancer. In fact, recent medical studies have found that cancerous tissues have a higher level of oxidation than healthy tissues, which suggests that the "clean up" mechanism intended to rid the body of harmful free radicals has been functioning inadequately.

Ground therapy has been shown to neutralize the negative effects of oxidative stress by eliminating free radicals in the body's bloodstream.

Ground therapy helps neutralize the impact of oxidative stress by eliminating the harmful free radicals that can overtax your body. As mentioned earlier, it does this by absorbing electrons from the earth so that your body's voltage is realigned in balance with the earth.

However, the story of why this all works is slightly more complicated. Electrons are negatively charged particles while free radicals are positively charged. This is why the free radicals, which lack an electron, are "attracted" to the electrons flowing into the body from the earth.

The earth's surface voltage is as close to neutral as possible, and is always less than 1.00 volt. An individual in a very healthy state will have a voltage as close to that of the earth as possible. But often this is not the case. When there are an excessive number of positively charged free radicals in the body, the voltage can often be above 1.00 volt, and in extreme cases may be as high as 3.00 or 4.00 volts.

And here is the crux of the matter: when we absorb electrons into our bodies, we are actually absorbing negative charge, which cancels out the positive charge created by free radicals. In fact, each unit of negative charge cancels out one unit of positive charge. The closer we can get to a neutral charge of 0.00 volts, the better for our bodies and our health. And this is exactly what ground therapy can accomplish.

Scientifically Proven Results

When ground therapy is used to clear out positively charged free radicals in the body, thereby balancing our overall voltage, the result is a reduction in our risk for chronic and degenerative illnesses, including cancer. Scientific research results confirm this.

One 2007 study, conducted by the Nature's Own Research Association, revealed that sleeping grounded is directly linked to a reduction of free radicals in the body. Not surprisingly, participants in the study slept better, felt better, and experienced more normal diurnal cortisol rhythms. The previously mentioned study by Ghaly and Teplitz which measured cortisol levels backs up this finding. One of the measurements that the researchers took in this study was of each subject's voltage before and after eight weeks of grounding. The table below, which shows the before and after voltage readings of each participant, provides concrete proof of the power of grounding to balance our electrical energy levels.

Subject	Voltage Before Grounding	Voltage After Grounding
1	3.940 V	0.003 V
2	1.470 V	0.001 V
3	2.700 V	0.004 V
4	1.200 V	0.002 V
5	2.700 V	0.005 V
6	1.670 V	0.005 V
7	5.950 V	0.008 V
8	3.940 V	0.008 V
9	3.750 V	0.010 V
10	2.300 V	0.009 V
11	5.980 V	0.020 V
12	3.640 V	0.006 V

As you can see, every single subject in this study experienced a dramatic decrease in voltage, which corresponds to an equally dramatic decrease in the level of cell-damaging free radicals in their systems. The fewer free radicals in our bloodstream, the healthier our cells, and the more easily we are able to carry out the standard tasks of our everyday lives. Ground therapy has a noticeable positive effect on the body, and that effect gives way to numerous trickle-down benefits, from boosting our energy levels to keeping us from aging so quickly.

> *The most reasonable hypothesis to explain the beneficial effects of earthing is that a direct earth connection enables...free electrons to flow from the earth to the body.* – Nature's Own Research Association

The Bottom Line on Ground Therapy and Cancer

We know that life is finite no matter how well we take care of ourselves, but we certainly want to avoid ending up with a compromised or diminished quality of life during the time we've been afforded. Striving to live cancer-free lives is one of the best ways to ensure a rich, healthy, and meaningful existence. And as you see from the information presented in this chapter, ground therapy offers a holistic, organic method for protecting ourselves from cancer. By rebalancing ourselves to the earth, we are actually allowing the earth to shield us in the way it was originally intended to do.

Chapter Seven

Heal Your Heart

People with heart disease and thick inflammatory blood (typical in patients with arterial disease and diabetes) may reap huge benefits from grounding themselves on a regular basis. Any time you can thin blood the consistency of ketchup to that of wine, as this simple experiment did, you minimize a significant risk factor for heart attack and stroke. This experiment showed that earthing can have this effect in a short period of time.

– Dr. Stephen Sinatra, Cardiologist

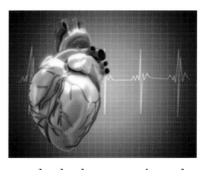

G round therapy plays a large role in preventing and reversing heart disease by regulating *heart rate variability* and *blood viscosity* (consistency). In addition, it helps calm the nervous system which safeguards the heart against the damaging effects of chronic stress. In an article about "going barefoot," Dr. Stephen Sinatra noted that the hippies of the 1960s were on to something revolutionary when they decided to kick off their shoes and get in touch with the earth. Although the research did not yet exist to prove why doing so contributed to "feeling groovy," we now know that grounding not only feels good, but is good for us as well. To fully appreciate the method by which ground therapy heals the heart, let's take a quick look at heart disease: what it is; what causes it; and what can happen to us if the heart disease epidemic goes on unchecked.

The Heart Disease Epidemic

Heart disease is the number one killer in the Western world, claiming more lives annually than cancer. The World Health Organization reports that in 2008, 25% of all deaths in the United States were caused by heart disease. Since then, that percentage has only increased. By 2030, 23.3 million people will die annually of cardiovascular diseases. Heart disease is on the increase not only in the Western world but in countries like China, where it was virtually non-existent until the second half of the 20th century.

According to a recent study compiled by the World Health Organization, 17.3 million people around the world die from heart disease every year. In other words, roughly 47,398 people are dying of cardiovascular illnesses like heart attacks and strokes *every single day*.

From these statistics, it's hard to ignore that heart disease has reached epidemic levels, especially in recent years. And it is clear that this epidemic is extremely costly, not only in terms of the massive suffering it causes to the individuals—and their families—who are afflicted, but also in terms of financial costs. In 2010, Americans spent $108,900,000,000 on heart disease alone—fighting it, trying to cure it, and trying to prevent it.

Why Our Hearts Are Breaking

Although it can manifest in many different ways, medical experts at the Mayo Clinic use the term "heart disease" to refer to damage caused by *atherosclerosis*—a buildup of fatty plaques in the arteries that causes them to harden.

Because the arterial system is responsible for carrying blood, nutrients, and oxygen from the heart to the rest of the body, atherosclerosis represents a serious problem that impacts virtually the whole body. Arteries that have grown thick and stiff with plaque 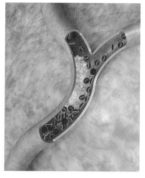 will restrict blood flow to the body's organs and tissues. Blood that is not constantly and freely flowing will begin to clot, and because atherosclerosis causes impeded blood flow, clots can form in the arteries. These clots will only restrict blood flow further, leading to heart attacks, strokes, and eventual death.

Like cancer, heart disease is considered to be a lifestyle disease. And as in the case of cancer and other lifestyle diseases, while we don't have control over every risk factor, there are a number that we *do* have significant choice about. The World Heart Federation has compiled a list that divides risk factors into two categories. *Modifiable risk factors* are facts about your life—such as lifestyle and environment choices—that are within your control and can be changed. This category also includes risk facts that from a theoretical perspective can be changed, but that are extremely difficult to change in practice. One such factor is living in poverty, which clearly causes many other health problems in addition to heart disease, but which may be beyond the power of individuals to alter. On the other hand, *non-modifiable* risk factors are those facets of your life that cannot be changed, such as age, gender, and genetic makeup.

The Tragic Toll of Heart Disease

Even where heart disease does not lead to death, it can seriously compromise one's quality of life, as well as place enormous financial and emotional burdens on other family members. That's why recognizing the signs of heart disease, and seeking medical advice if you experience any warning signs, is especially important. According to researchers at the esteemed Mayo Clinic, the symptoms of cardiovascular illness typically include:

- Chest pain (angina)
- Shortness of breath
- Pain or numbness in legs and arms
- Weakness or coldness in legs and arms
- A fluttering in your chest (arrhythmia)
- A racing heartbeat (tachycardia)
- A slowed heartbeat (bradycardia)
- Lightheadedness
- Dizziness
- Fainting

Identifying these symptoms and seeking treatment is half the battle. The other half is focused on preventative measures to ensure that you stay healthy in the first place—such as ground therapy.

How Ground Therapy Heals Your Heart

According to cardiologist Dr. Stephen Sinatra, ground therapy benefits the heart in numerous ways. The first is by regulating something called heart rate variability (HRV), which can be described as the beat-to-beat alterations in heart rate. Individuals with a high variability rate are more likely to be in better health and have higher levels of fitness. Individuals with a lower HRV, on the other hand, are typically stressed out or fatigued. People with a lower HRV are less able to "go with the flow" when it comes to stress, and are thus more likely to get hypertension and cardiac disease. This is because many of the hormones produced during the stress response are highly damaging to the human heart, especially if produced to excess, as is the case with chronic stress.

The second way that ground therapy helps our hearts is by balancing the body's nervous system. When we ground ourselves, we are regulating our *autonomic nervous system* (ANS). The ANS is made up of two branches—the sympathetic branch and the parasympathetic branch—that govern many systems of the body, including the circulatory system. When we are under stress, the sympathetic nervous system springs into action, triggering the fight or flight response, which sends our blood pressure up and our hearts pounding. Ground therapy has been shown to calm the activity of the sympathetic nervous system, which quiets the stress response. Or to put it another way, balancing the ANS leads to an increase in HRV, which leads directly to better heart health.

Improvements in HRV that occur as a result of ground therapy always lead to a reduction in sympathetic activity and a balance of the ANS— and ultimately, then, a healthier heart.

The third way that ground therapy helps heal our hearts is by reducing *blood viscosity*. Simply stated, blood viscosity is a measure of the thickness of our blood. Medical research has linked moderate to high blood viscosity with cardiovascular disease, and some individuals have even developed a cardiovascular disorder called hyper viscosity syndrome. Highly viscous blood can lead to plaque and platelet buildup, as well as atherosclerosis.

Dr. Stephen Sinatra's research has revealed that blood samples from individuals who have been grounded for as little as *40 minutes* tend to be less viscous than blood samples from individuals who have not been grounded at all. Individuals whose blood tested as highly viscous before grounding will often show dramatic improvement after grounding, with their blood samples showing far less blood cell, plaque, and platelet coagulation. These and other scientifically proven findings have profound implications for the role of ground therapy in helping to prevent or reverse risk factors associated with cardiovascular disease.

Scientifically Proven Results

A study conducted by Gaétan Chevalier, PhD, for the *Journal of Alternative and Complementary Medicine*, found evidence that indirectly links ground therapy with heart health. The study measured the electrical conductance of the skin. The amount of skin conductance varies with the skin's moisture level, so that a high level indicates that the body's sweat glands have been activated by the sympathetic nervous system. In other words, the body is in a state of emergency arousal and its fight or flight response has been triggered. By contrast, a lower skin conductance usually corresponds to a calmly functioning sympathetic nervous system, which means that the ANS is balanced and the body is not in a state of constant stress. After just 40 minutes of grounding patients experienced a reduction in skin conductance, which indicates that the arousal level of the sympathetic nervous system had decreased.

Another study conducted by Drs. Gaétan Chevalier, Stephen Sinatra, James Oschman, and Richard Delany confirms the results of the Chevalier study mentioned above. The research findings, published in the *Journal of Alternative and Complementary Medicine*, revealed that earthing dramatically reduces levels of blood viscosity in the human body. During this study 10 healthy adults (aged 42 to 63) were grounded for two hours, with blood samples taken both before and afterwards. Tests were conducted on the samples to evaluate a number of factors including *zeta potential* and *red blood cell* (RBC) *clumping*.

Zeta potential is a way of measuring the mobility of blood cells within the blood stream. A higher zeta potential reflects more space between the cells, as well as lower viscosity and lower resistance to blood flow. Zeta potential is a negative charge, and works on a relatively simple scientific principle: like charges oppose like. In other words, two negative charges will repel each other.

Before grounding, subjects had lower zeta potentials and more RBC clumping. After grounding, however, their zeta potentials had increased two- and even three-fold. RBC clumping was also greatly diminished, which shows that the flood of electrons absorbed from the earth had caused healthy repelling charges among RBCs in the bloodstream. When the RBCs were repelled, they tended to stop coagulating and clumping together. In turn, this allowed the blood to move more quickly and freely through the subjects' arteries—an important key to cardiovascular health.

These results and others demonstrate that grounding is effective at lowering the viscosity of the blood and diminishing the risk of developing cardiovascular disease.

The Bottom Line on Ground Therapy and Heart Health

No matter who you are, where you live, or how you live, your life has probably been touched by heart disease. Chances are you know someone who suffers from the tragic and frightening consequences of cardiovascular disease, or maybe you yourself are afflicted with it. Either way, heart disease presents a threat to our lives on a daily basis, and the risk only increases as we age. But ground therapy represents new hope for protecting ourselves from cardiovascular problems. And, even where mobility and breathing are impacted by already-present heart disease, ground therapy is appropriate because it requires very little physical effort and is so simple to do.

Taking even a few minutes a day to become grounded and in tune with the earth will help stabilize the body's electrical charge, which results in the strengthening of our arteries and our heart muscles, the reduction in the thickness of our blood and a whole host of other benefits as well. Ground therapy truly can heal our hearts!

Chapter Eight

Better Sleep for a Longer, Healthier Life

Aside from the risk of death in extreme sleep deprivation, there are clearly numerous reasons that we should get enough rest to minimize the risks associated with inadequate sleep. We imperil our health when we fail to do so. – Dr. Brandon Peters, M.D.

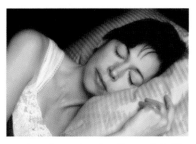

Sleep may seem like one of the most natural things in the world, and sleeping well and waking up rested and refreshed is a wonderful feeling. But for many people bedtime represents the start of a nightly struggle to get to sleep, to stay asleep, and to clock enough hours of rest. For some, the struggle originates even before bedtime, because a too-busy, over-full schedule can make it difficult to carve out the seven to eight hours a night that we need for adequate rest. Others manage to set aside the required time, but find it almost impossible to fall asleep, or toss and turn all night in an interrupted sleep pattern that is anything but restful

Of course, everyone has the occasional night when sleep is elusive, but a surprising number of people suffer from sleep disorders that prevent them from getting the rest that is so critical for rejuvenating our bodies and keeping us healthy. For those individuals, ground therapy can prove invaluable, because sleeping grounded helps reduce the chemical compounds that promote activity and wakefulness and induces the deep state of calm and relaxation that makes sleep possible. And these benefits are especially important for those recovering from illness, whose bodies are already under an unusually high stress load.

I've had a grounding wire hooked up to me for about two weeks now and wow! My sleep since my illness has never been better. – Test subject

The effects of ground therapy for sleep regulation are easiest to appreciate in the context of the sleep deprivation epidemic itself—including what causes it and why it is so hard to fight.

The Sleep Deprivation Epidemic

Sleep deprivation is not a benign condition, and neither is it rare. In fact, sleep disorders are so common that the United States Centers for Disease Control and Prevention (CDC) characterizes the problem of insufficient sleep as a public health issue of epidemic proportions. In part, this is because inadequate sleep impacts not only on our energy levels, but is linked to a number of chronic diseases that impact negatively on every aspect of our lives.

Sleep is increasingly recognized as important to public health .... Persons experiencing sleep insufficiency are also more likely to suffer from chronic diseases such as hypertension, diabetes, depression, and obesity, as well as from cancer, increased mortality, and reduced quality of life and productivity. – United States Centers for Disease Control and Prevention

But another part of the problem is that people tend to underestimate the importance of a good night's sleep. In our over-scheduled, hyper-busy lifestyles, one of the first activities to be sacrificed when we are short on time is sleep. After rushing around all day, we often find that there's still more we need to do before we can go to bed, so we push our bedtimes back later and later. Then in the morning, we often find that we have to get up early to fit in the things we simply couldn't complete the night before, and then rush to get to work on time. This pattern is fairly common is our modern society; the more responsibilities we have, the less sleep we are inclined to get. But ironically, in order to stay healthy the pattern should actually be *reversed*; the more we have to do, the more sleep we need. And when we consider that lack of sleep is often accompanied by insomniac worry and stress, it is no wonder that experts believe that we are an "under-slept" nation burning the candle at both ends, and effectively running on empty.

And it's also little wonder that so many people suffer from health issues related to sleep. According to a new study from the American Academy of Sleep Medicine, one in five adults in the United States regularly experiences moderate to severe daytime sleepiness. The leader of this study, Dr. Maurice Ohayon, professor of psychiatry at Stanford, says that these statistics reveal that the occurrence of daytime sleepiness is much higher in individuals in America than in Europe, which signals that it is becoming a significant health issue. The study, which surveyed 8,937 people in Texas, New York, and California in an effort to identify the prevalence of consistent patterns of sleep loss across all groups, came to a stunning conclusion: Americans are so exhausted that we are more or less *sleepwalking* our way through our daily activities.

Enemies of Sleep

Electronics are making it very enticing to stay up later. You have 500 cable channels, 24/7 entertainment and technologies, video gaming available around the clock. How bad something is for you depends on the extent to which it is captivating you and tempting you not to sleep. – Dr. Charles Czeisler

You may be well acquainted with some of the culprits of sleep loss—daily stress, too much work, insufficient or unhealthy meals—but there are others that may surprise you. Dr. Charles A. Czeisler, director of sleep medicine at Harvard's Brigham & Women's Hospital in Boston,

110

recently co-authored a National Sleep Foundation survey that identified electronics usage as the *number one* culprit for sleep loss and disrupted sleep.

One reason that our electronic gadgets lead to sleep loss is that they are so entertaining! Gaming, watching television, and surfing the net can tempt us to stay up "just a little while longer" which often ends up being hours later than we should. But further exacerbating the problem is the fact that these gadgets bombard our bodies with EMF stimulation. And added to the threat EMFs constitute for our health, many of our electronics also emit light pollution, which stimulates our bodies to remain awake by preventing the release of sleep-enhancing hormones such as melatonin. The overall impact of modern living—coupled with our love of our electronics—is that sleep health is at risk. And as we saw earlier, the number of people affected is not only vast, it is also growing. A full 64% of the respondents in Dr. Czeisler's study said that they woke up at least once during the night, and 61% said they woke up in the morning feeling un-refreshed at least a few times a week. This means that those in the 61% are experiencing the after-effects of sleep deprivation or disruption almost as often as half the time.

And it appears that electronics usage is one of the factors involved in their sleep problems. In fact, about 95% of the survey participants said that they use some form of electronic device such as a laptop, cell phone, or television before going to bed. Although we often think of activities like texting, surfing the Internet, or playing video games as things that help us "unwind" after a long day, the converse is actually true. These devices put our minds and bodies into a hyper-alert and over-stimulated state, which is clearly counterproductive to sleep. Add to that the harmful impact of EMFs on our bodies, and we shouldn't be surprised that when we finally do go to bed, neither mind nor body is in the relaxed state necessary for sleep.

Although we've discussed EMFs in general, a special mention is warranted with respect to household EMFs, which are emitted from the technologies in our homes. In 1995, a study by the National Institute of Environmental Health Sciences and the US Department of Energy found that daily exposure to household EMFs can produce unnaturally weak currents between human cells, which skews the body's voltage upwards and out of the neutral range typical of the voltage of the earth.

Today everyone is physically stressed, their muscles are tense, back and joint pain are the norm, and most do not sleep well. These conditions all relate to excess stimulation of the nervous system and/or interference with the biochemical communication between cells. – Clint Ober

If you are living and sleeping in a modern home, you are being exposed to household EMFs on a constant basis. The electronics we use not only over-stimulating the mind, but the ANS (*autonomic nervous system*) as well. When we bombard our bodies with EMFs, we are essentially interrupting crucial communications among cells and

activating the stress response. The resulting overstimu-
lation of our nervous systems directly interferes with our
ability to get restful sleep. Not surprisingly, this can lead
to a state in which our bodies are physically stressed as
well. And as you probably know, physical stress acts as a
barrier to restful sleep—or even getting to sleep at all—
which sets up an unhealthy cycle of exhaustion feeding
stress, which in turn fuels further exhaustion

The Devastating Effects of Sleep Deprivation

We may all be familiar with the short-term side effects
of a night or two of sleep deprivation—grogginess, drowsi-
ness, confusion, impaired memory function. If our sleep
deprivation is short-lived, we can catch up on sleep the
following night and alleviate our symptoms immediately.
But when we are living and working in stressful environments that do not allow us to get sufficient amounts of
sleep over the long term, sleep deprivation may become
chronic, with devastating results.

Sleep is widely understood to be one of the body's most
crucial restorative processes. Recent studies have found
that sleep is essential for a number of reasons. First, it
allows for the process of cellular renewal to take place.
This process protects us from disease and keeps us looking
and feeling young by replacing injured muscle tissue and
destroying dead cells throughout the body. Sleep is also
the best time for the brain to process and archive
information (including memories) so that our minds and
cognitive processes stay sharp. In addition, the REM
(rapid eye movement) phase of the sleep cycle, which

coincides with dreaming, has been shown to activate areas of the brain associated with learning. In other words, sleep doesn't just refresh our energy levels for another day, it repairs and protects our bodies, our minds, and our health. And, as you might well imagine, the health consequences of sleep deprivation can be quite severe.

Insulin Resistance

When we don't sleep enough, our body's blood sugar can become dis-regulated, peaking in the middle of the night and saturating our bloodstreams with glucose. This can lead to chronic conditions such as Type 2 diabetes.

Hormonal Dis-regulation

When we sleep, our bodies are able to regulate the hormones *leptin* and *ghrelin*, which control the body's hunger response. In a healthy body, leptin (which signals that we are full) and ghrelin (which signals that we are hungry) are typically released three times a day, which corresponds to the three-meal-a-day pattern most of us follow. In the sleep-deprived body, however, leptin and ghrelin are released more frequently, and at extremely erratic times. Sometimes we will be awakened by hunger, or find ourselves hungry after eating a full meal. The fact that our hunger cues are disordered can lead to overeating and ultimately to obesity.

Heart Disease

As previously stated, sleep deprivation is closely linked with the body's stress response. When we are stressed out, we enter into the hyper-alert state of fight or flight, which causes the ANS to work strenuously. When our ANS is working overtime, needless to say it is extremely difficult to fall asleep—and to stay asleep. These sleep difficulties result in more stress, which only exacerbates the problem. When the body is in a state of chronic stress, complications like increased blood pressure and viscosity are more likely to arise, which increases the potential of cardiovascular conditions like hypertension, heart attack, and stroke.

Depression

Depression is a debilitating mental illness that often results in *anhedonia*, or a sense of apathy about the activities you once enjoyed. For a chronically depressed person, work, hobbies, and sex can all seem meaningless and not worth the effort. Lack of sleep has been directly linked to depression, and for a good reason; sleep is when we process the events of the day, learn from them, and then store them away in our memories. If we cannot process our experiences in such a way, our lives begin to seem like a series of disconnected events. This lack of continuity can lead to feelings of hopelessness, confusion, and depression.

Are You Sleep Deprived?

Knowing that sleep deprivation is dangerous for your health is one thing. But how do you recognize the signals of sleep deprivation? According to sleep experts, the nine key signs of sleep deprivation are:

- Short-term memory loss
- Inability to concentrate

- Increased appetite

- Fuzzy or blurry vision

- Impaired decision-making

- Diminished motor skills

- Relationship troubles

- Mood swings

If you are experiencing *three or more* of these signs—and especially if you experience them on a regular basis—you may be sleep deprived. Recognizing that sleep deprivation is the cause of your symptoms is actually good news, because it allows you to take action before your sleep problems lead to serious medical issues. And perhaps you've already suspected that inadequate sleep is a problem for you, and tried to address it by making an extra effort to get more sleep. But if so, you may be like many others who have discovered that despite your efforts, sleep remains elusive. And that is where ground therapy comes in. Because ground therapy has worked for many people when everything else they've tried has failed!

How Ground Therapy
Fights Sleep Deprivation

EMFs are keeping us awake by over-stimulating our minds and our nervous systems, and if or when we do manage to sleep at all, they disrupt important inter-cellular communications, which in turn disrupts the body's processes of healing. And this chaotic state of the human body is brought about by a lack of connection with the earth. But ground therapy reverses the chaos by preventing EMFs from interfering with the communication among cells, which not only will allow you to get the rest you need, but as we've seen, also helps bring about a radical reduction in pain and inflammation.

In modern times, humans have insulated themselves from contact with the earth by wearing synthetic soled shoes and living in homes that elevate the body above the earth. Consequently, humans are no longer naturally grounded and now the body becomes charged with static electricity and radiated electric fields, which can create unnatural weak electric currents within the body. Loss of connection with the natural ground allows extraneous electricity to interfere with and stress the normal bioelectrical activities of the body, thereby interfering with natural health and sleep. – Clint Ober

When we ground ourselves, we protect ourselves from the static electricity and radiated electric fields that comprise harmful EMFs. When we are grounded, we are able to protect ourselves from EMFs by absorbing the earth's electrons into our own systems, thus reducing the voltage of our bodies. Once protected from the radiated and dangerous EMFs, our bodies are able to carry out their biochemical processes—facilitated by inter-cellular communication—without interference.

What does all this mean for our overall health? It's relatively simple, really. The more of the earth's electrons we have in our bodies, the better our bodies function. With respect to sleep disorders, which are intimately linked with stress, this means that both stress levels and length and quality of sleep improve. In other words, ground therapy fights sleep deprivation by dramatically reducing the levels of certain chemicals in our bodies that have been linked to stress and lack of sleep.

Scientifically Proven Results

Since reduction in stress levels and reduction in sleep deprivation go hand in hand, ground therapy studies showing a reduction in stress levels tend to show an improvement in sleeping habits. One such study, conducted by Dr. Karol Sokal and Dr. Pawel Sokal, found that sleeping grounded had a tremendous positive influence on the biological systems that regulate sleep and relaxation. In an article entitled *"Earthing the Human Body Influences Physiologic Processes"* which was published in the *Journal of Alternative and Complementary Medicine*, the doctors described their findings. One of the most statistically significant was that blood glucose levels in subjects who were grounded decreased.

During the study, 12 adults (ages of 42 to 58) were separated into two groups and instructed to go about their daily activities. The only difference between the two groups was that one was continually grounded for 72 hours, while the other was not. Blood glucose levels were measured at the beginning of the trial, again after 24 hours, and once more after 72 hours. While the readings of the ungrounded group remained relatively stable and unchanged during the 72 hour period, the group that had been grounded showed a *significant* reduction in blood glucose levels.

Why is this finding so important? And what does a reduction in blood glucose mean for overall health? High blood glucose is an indicator that our stress response is working overtime. Glucose is produced to meet the energy needs of the body. The more energy our bodies anticipate burning, the more glucose is produced. But if the energy demands of the body do not use up all the glucose produced, the excess glucose level in the bloodstream can lead to future chronic health problems like obesity and Type 2 diabetes.

But high blood glucose can also cause problems in the immediate term. Excess glucose in our blood may cause reactions such as pounding hearts, sweating, and racing thoughts. It's not difficult to see why these reactions would interfere with the ability to sleep. On the other hand, reduced blood glucose usually means that the body has entered the relaxed state that is conducive to sleep. It stands to reason, then, that those who sleep grounded typically sleep better than they did before they were grounded.

Another important result the doctors Karol obtained was a noticeable improvement in thyroid function in adults who slept grounded overnight. Twelve patients between 34 and 60 years old were divided into two groups: a grounded group and an ungrounded group. Levels of thyroid-stimulating hormone (TSH) and the thyroid hormones T3 and T4 were measured before the participants went to sleep at night, and again in the morning after they awoke. These measurements can give realms of important information about the health of the thyroid, and how well it is functioning.

TSH stimulates the thyroid to perform its duties by producing T3 and T4. The T3 hormone has been referred to as the "gas pedal" of the body; it stimulates our metabolisms and gets our bodies running. The T4 hormone is a "stored" version of T3—it gets converted to T3 when the need arises.

Having high levels of T3 is often a sign of hyperthyroid syndrome—it means your body is working in overdrive. The symptoms of *hyperthyroid syndrome* correlate closely with the symptoms of stress—increased heart rate, anxiety, weight loss, and difficulty sleeping.

When your body has an excess of T3, it is probably working in an overstressed state. A decrease in T3—combined with an increase in TSH and T4—means your thyroid is returning to normal, and your body is entering a relaxed state.

In the subjects who slept grounded, the levels of TSH and T4 were both increased, while the amount of T3 decreased. These results are important for human health because our thyroids have a significant impact on the regulation of crucial biological processes in our bodies. In fact, the thyroid gland is involved in pretty much every bodily process. It increases our basal metabolic rate, facilitates protein synthesis, regulates growth and development, metabolizes carbohydrates, and stabilizes body temperature. All this from a tiny gland that usually weighs less than 30 grams!

A properly-functioning thyroid is also an important factor in getting a good night's sleep. In a healthy person, the thyroid will prevent the body from metabolizing glucose too quickly, so that you aren't awoken by hunger in the middle of the night and can enjoy your full quota of *uninterrupted sleep.*

Overall, the enormous value of this study is that it proves conclusively that grounded subjects—even if they are only grounded for a single night—show a reduction in stress- and anxiety-causing chemicals in their blood serum, which leads to an improvement in the ability to relax and fall asleep, and to avoid sleep interruptions.

The Bottom Line on Ground Therapy and Better Sleep

The key to getting good sleep is relaxation, and we all know that stress is a barrier to relaxation. When the human body is healthy and functioning as intended, it produces chemical compounds at specific times throughout the day to regulate important physiological processes such as sleep, wakefulness, and hunger. But when our body's systems are out of whack, it produces these compounds at irregular times, preventing us from getting the restorative rest we need. Ground therapy can help us get back into a healthy balance again by reducing the stress-producing chemicals in our blood so that we can fall asleep. And when we sleep grounded, we sleep deeply and uninterrupted because the earth's electrons are removing the harmful chemicals from our bloodstreams that would otherwise cause us to wake up too soon.

Chapter Nine

Supercharge Your Immunity, Heal Autoimmune Disorders, and End Chronic Disease

When the immune system is overworked or weak due to chronic stress, poor nutrition, or exposure to chemical/ environmental toxicities ... it is less effective at removing toxic and mutated cells or harmful pathogens. The resulting consequences can be severe, leading to the development of chronic illnesses that can be debilitating. – Dr. Aaron Hoo

By living disconnected from the earth, we cut ourselves off from our planet's immunity-boosting properties, while throwing our bodies into a state of imbalance and vulnerability. As a result, our immune systems become compromised and weakened—and we are prone to developing debilitating disease.

Compromised immunity is associated with a long and rather frightening list of potential health consequences, including chronic diseases ranging from cancer to multiple sclerosis to Alzheimer's—and many more. But when we reconnect with the earth, the immunological effects, including protection from chronic disease, are measurable and profound.

Ground therapy boosts our immunity by shielding us from harmful EMFs that can interrupt intercellular communication and decrease immune response. As mentioned previously, renowned integrative doctor and ground therapy enthusiast Dr. Joseph Mercola explains that this shielding occurs when the human body derives extra electrons from the earth.

Your immune system functions optimally when your body has an adequate supply of electrons, which are easily and naturally obtained by barefoot contact with the earth. – Dr. Joseph Mercola

The High Price of Weak Immunity

Our immune systems keep us healthy by protecting us from toxins that could do serious harm to our bodies. Without our immune systems, we would be virtually helpless in the world, completely defenseless against even the most benign bacterium. A robust immune system is the key to a long and healthy life because it not only protects us from developing acute illness from such things as the common cold, but it also cushions us from feeling the full and debilitating effects of pain. But safeguarding us against chronic health issues and serious diseases such as cancer is the immune system's stellar role.

Individuals with disorders that compromise and weaken their immune systems, such as AIDS, are at a significantly higher risk for developing chronic diseases than individuals whose immune system is strong. According to a study in the *Journal of the American Medical Association*, male AIDS patients were found to have an 11 times higher risk of developing Hodgkin's disease, were 3 times as likely to develop lip cancer, and twice as likely to develop some form of testicular cancer. This is because a radically weakened immune system has a much more difficult time destroying unhealthy cells.

However, the absence of an *obvious* immune disorder is not a reason to assume that your immune system is functioning optimally. This is crucial information, and it is well worth repeating. The fact that an immune system illness is not obvious does not guarantee that your immune system is uncompromised, nor does it mean that if your immune system is healthy at present, that it will remain that way.

Otherwise "healthy" people are compromising their immune systems every day. Our modern lifestyles expose us to more toxins than any previous population in human history. When you consider the overwhelming cascade of toxins that engulf us daily from cigarettes, polluted air, chemically altered food, and EMFs, it soon becomes clear just how heavy a burden our lifestyles put on our immune systems. Over an extended period of time, our over-whelmed immune systems start to fall behind in the task of protecting us. When that happens, toxins quickly gain the upper hand by killing off healthy cells more quickly than our bodies can repair them.

If this barrage of toxins continues for a long enough period of time our immune systems simply start to shut down altogether, which leaves us prone to the quick and unimpeded development of chronic disease. In an editorial in the *Journal of Complementary and Alternative Medicine*, ground therapy expert Dr. James L. Oschman explored the relationship between immunological deficiency and chronic disease. Since chronic inflammation and compromised immunity go hand-in-hand, he suspected that an improvement in immunity would result in the overall reduction of chronic disease. His research revealed links between compromised immunity and the following chronic conditions:

- Alzheimer's disease

- Asthma

- Atherosclerosis

- Bowel disorders

- Cancer

- Chronic obstructive pulmonary disease

- Cirrhosis of the liver

- Cystic fibrosis

- Diabetes

- Meningitis

- Multiple sclerosis

- Osteoporosis

- Prostate cancer

- Psoriasis

- Rheumatoid arthritis

This is a sobering list, and it not only illustrates why strong immunity is so critical, but also why it is so important that we understand what we can do to combat the process of immune system degradation. Doing so will not only protect our overall health but will also help us avoid the enormously costly repercussions (personal, social, and financial) that can negatively impact our lives when chronic disease becomes our reality.

Many chronic diseases are lifelong conditions, and impact the quality of life not only of those suffering from the diseases, but also of their family members, caregivers, and others. Stemming the growth in the enormous costs related to chronic disease has become a major public priority, as the government, employers, and consumers increasingly struggle to keep up. – Dr. James Oschman

A Deadly Pairing: The Terrible Link Between Compromised Immunity and Inflammation

Weak immunity is directly related to the major culprit behind virtually all chronic disease—chronic inflammation. As explained fully in Chapter Two, chronic inflammation is a condition that causes the immune system to continuously mount a response to foreign toxins in the body. In the process, an excess of free radicals are released, which if left unchecked will eventually begin attacking healthy cells.

After working non-stop for so long the immune system ultimately becomes overtaxed and exhausted, losing its ability to fight off legitimate infections. As this endlessly negative cycle continues, the chronically inflamed body essentially destroys itself from within.

One significant symptom of chronic inflammation that is brought about by immunological weakness is pain. According to a ground therapy study on chronic pain conducted by Clint Ober, increased levels of free radicals in the body can cause oxidative stress, which in turn can cause chronic pain. Muscles, ligaments, and joints are most likely to bear the brunt—and feel the acute pain—of oxidative stress. Free radicals eat away at the healthy tissue of our joints, muscles, and ligaments, limiting our freedom of movement and causing chronic pain. Chronic pain of this sort can seriously compromise our independence and quality of life.

In addition to pain, constant overproduction of free radicals by the immune system creates the perfect conditions for inflammatory-related diseases to take hold. Chronic health issues like arthritis, arteriosclerosis, heart attack, Type 2 diabetes, lupus, multiple sclerosis, asthma, and inflammatory bowel disease are now shown to be directly linked with poor immune function.

And finally, a compromised immune system leaves us highly susceptible to colds and other viruses and illnesses. When our immune systems have been weakened by stress, toxins, and EMFs, we become more prone to contracting a virus or cold, and less able to fight them off. Although catching a cold or flu may seem fairly minor in comparison to the risk of developing a serious chronic disease, when your immune system is compromised the costs of doing so are heightened. For instance, you can expect that your recovery period will take an extra week, which might represent the difference between receiving a promotion and being terminated. This is just an example, of course, but the point is that every extra day that we must spend recovering is time lost, time taken away from our normal lives. And regardless of what our normal lives look like, being laid up with illness after illness robs us of vitality and joy.

All of these implications make it supremely important to recognize that the following symptoms may indicate a weakened or compromised immune system:

- Chronic and frequent infections

- Recurring infections

- Developing new allergies

- Constant fatigue

- Insomnia

- Depression

- Dark circles under the eyes

- Poor response to treatment for infections

- Delayed or incomplete recovery from illness

- Cuts or wounds that will not heal

Recognizing these symptoms early and taking action to strengthen your immune system immediately are two important steps in the process of fighting back against a weakened immune system. Most important, however, is seeking a permanent path to recovery. And that's where the revolutionary science of ground therapy comes in.

How Ground Therapy Fights Weak Immunity

As mentioned, Clint Ober has shown that free radical levels are increased by exposure to EMFs. We live and work in environments that are highly charged and irradiated; when we are exposed to such radiation, our bodies adapt by becoming "dipole antennae" that attract the force field of EMFs. Simply put, our bodies acquire a charge, and that charge attracts other charges. This only serves to increase the amount of free radicals in our bodies, further damaging our tissues and overtaxing our immune systems.

Exposure to electromagnetic fields between 50-60 Hz increases concentrations of free radicals in the body, lengthens their lifespan, and can lead to serious damage in the body.

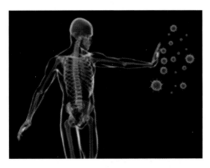

When we ground ourselves, by contrast, our bodies acquire the natural electrical voltage of the earth, eliminating the dipole antennae effect. Not only does this prevent the further proliferation of free radicals, it actually *reverses* their effect on the body. And as we have seen, individuals suffering from compromised immune systems and chronic pain have overwhelmingly reported that their symptoms improved or were eradicated altogether after just *one night* of sleeping grounded.

The extra electrons absorbed from the earth when we are grounded have the added effect of improving intercellular communication, allowing the body's biological systems to run more smoothly. The result is that T-cells can communicate better and thus will have an easier time identifying what is and is not a foreign toxin. This accuracy makes it immeasurably easier for your immune system to do the job nature intended and fight off real threats and infections.

For instance, thyroid cells that can communicate freely with one another will be able to produce the correct amounts of crucial hormones, including TSH, T3, and T4. Endocrine cells will better understand how much ghrelin (the hunger hormone) your body needs. With all the cells buffered by electrons against harmful free radicals, debilitating conditions such as immune weakness and chronic inflammation will swiftly become things of the past.

Scientifically Proven Results

The most significant results in favor of ground therapy's dramatic positive effect on the immune system come from the Sokal study mentioned earlier. This study is notable for its findings regarding the ability of grounded subjects to regulate their sleep schedules, but it is also notable for its findings on the immune systems of grounded patients.

One part of the Sokal study involved exploring the effects of grounding on subjects' immune response to a typhoid vaccine. For this purpose, 32 healthy volunteers aged 19 to 23 were given the vaccine. All participants spent the next two days ungrounded. On the third day, half of the group was grounded, and blood samples from all participants were taken the following day. The blood samples taken from the grounded individuals were found to have considerably higher amounts of immune cells such as T cells, globulins, and albumins when compared with samples from the ungrounded individuals. This indicates that the effect of grounding was to support a robust immunological response to the vaccine, which was con-current with a decrease of toxins in the blood of the grounded individuals.

To put it simply, sleeping grounded strengthens the immune system, protecting it from EMFs and allowing it to accurately identify and neutralize threatening toxins.

Another remarkable result of ground therapy is its reduction—and virtual elimination—of pain in patients suffering from disorders caused by chronic inflammation (as discussed in Chapter Three). In Clint Ober's study of the effects of ground therapy on chronic pain, every single subject experienced a reduction in pain as a result of sleeping grounded. The subjects, who were suffering from a diverse array of muscle and joint pains, were universally consistent in their positive results after only a few nights of sleeping grounded. Grounding was shown to alleviate or altogether eliminate the following types of chronic pain:

- Neck stiffness
- Leg and foot cramps
- Arthritis
- Carpal tunnel
- Menstrual cramps
- Headaches
- Gas pain and constipation
- TMJ
- Back pain
- Joint pain

The Bottom Line on Ground Therapy and Better Immunity

Ground therapy is beneficial to the immune system because it allows our bodies to maintain *homeostasis*, which is defined as a property of a system that has a regulated internal environment. In the case of the complex system of the human body, the "regulated internal environment" would be achieved when all the body's systems are communicating with each other and working together in harmony. This harmony allows the immune system to do its job of protecting our health properly, which makes yet another good reason to join the ground therapy revolution.

Chapter Ten

The Revolution Ahead

All truth passes through three stages. First, it is ridiculed. Second, it is violently opposed. Third, it is accepted as being self-evident. – Arthur Schopenhauer

The reason we've lost touch with the earth is because our "modern" lifestyle insulates us from the earth's healing properties. We live indoors, work indoors, wear plastic-soled shoes, and often have little opportunity to walk barefoot outdoors safely. While convenient and practical, this lifestyle is also artificial. And as we continue to live in ways that could be described as increasingly *unnatural,* in the sense of being distanced from nature itself, the human body (which is, after all, part of nature) inevitably rebels in some way or other. We can see this in the fact that diabetes, heart disease, and cancer are not natural conditions of the human body. Rather, they are diseases that humankind has acquired as a result of living our insulated and disconnected modern lives.

> *Health is natural. And part of being naturally healthy and functioning optimally appears to involve connectedness to the earth. Being disconnected seems both unnatural and unhealthy... We live on our planet, but we have insulated ourselves from it, and at great cost.* – Clint Ober

Chronic disease and its causes—such as chronic inflammation, stress, and fatigue—are all consequences of living in a way that is out of touch with the earth, so that our bodies' electron balance is thrown out of whack. But as we have seen throughout this book, when we ground ourselves in harmony with the earth our bodies are able to correct their electron deficiencies and revert to their healthy, natural states.

> *People have been led to believe that national health insurance, more doctors, and greater use of high-cost hospital-based technologies will improve health. Unfortunately, none of them will.*
>
> – Dr. John Knowles

The need for a new healing modality like ground therapy is more important now than ever. In the near future, almost 80 million American baby boomers will turn 65. As we have seen, an increased risk of chronic disease is already associated with aging, but if we assume that the majority of these baby boomers have been living 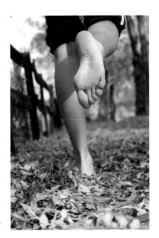 "typical" modern lives (disconnected from nature and the earth) then it is clear that the risk of developing a life-threatening illness in late middle age increases exponentially. And unfortunately Americans are not the only ones facing a significant health decline. According to a recent report by the World Health Organization, chronic disease has been ravaging countries the world over. In 2008, chronic, non-communicable diseases (lifestyle diseases) were responsible for the deaths of more than *36 million people* worldwide. About a quarter of those deaths — roughly 9 million—were classified as "premature," meaning that they occurred before individuals had reached the age of 60. Although it is true that many of these premature deaths occurred in developing countries that could not provide their patients with the appropriate healthcare, first-world countries are beginning to experience an upsurge in premature deaths as well. The United States is at the forefront of this group, because our healthcare system is strained to the breaking point. We are overwhelmed by sickness and running out of money to pay for everyone's recovery.

> *Instead of focusing on health insurance, we need to emphasize health assurance.* – Clint Ober

This means, that we must make take matters into our own hands to the extent that we can. Joseph D. Beasley M.D., and Jerry Swift, M.A., authors of *The Kellogg Report: The Impact of Nutrition, Environment, and Lifestyle on the Health of Americans*, concur, saying that it is now time to take responsibility for our own health. This involves making the maintenance of our health a priority, and taking preventative measures against chronic illness.

And as this book has demonstrated in numerous ways, one of the most effective ways to do so is with ground therapy. Unlike undergoing chemotherapy or having coronary bypass surgery, ground therapy is easy and inexpensive. In many cases, ground therapy is even entirely free—all you need to do is spend some time outside barefoot. If you have access to a safe, clean outdoor area, the inconvenience of going outside without shoes is well worth the payoff of preventing chronic disease and keeping healthcare bills down.

If walking barefoot outdoors is not an option, or if you—like many—are already suffering symptoms of chronic inflammation and other health problems, then more powerful options such as easy-to-use conductive devices offer a powerful and realistic solution. In either case, ground therapy offers us a mode of self-care that will help restore the natural, biological balance that has been lost to our poor lifestyle habits. Granted, we cannot go back in time and undo those lifestyle habits, but we can rely on the earth to reverse the negative effects—and to heal us.

Self-care is the only effective way to ensure good health and a longer, fuller life. While there is a crying need for reforms of the healthcare system, the most needed reform of all is our own attitudes. We patients must become activists for our own health.
– Joseph D. Beasley M.D., and Jerry Swift, M.A.

The Astounding Positive Impact
of Ground Therapy

Given the nearly miraculous things that ground therapy can do for your health, it wouldn't be an overstatement to say that the discovery of ground therapy is of the same magnitude as the invention of the telephone, the television, and the computer. Each of these technologies changed the world and it seems almost inconceivable to think of living our lives in the same way we did before their invention. Ground therapy has at least as much potential to impact our world as profoundly as these technologies have, if not more. Clint Ober believes that ground therapy has the power to change how people live. It is both evolutionary and revolutionary, in that it invites us to take a new perspective on our lives and on our health.

And it has the potential to entirely transform the way medicine is practiced as well. For one thing, as a healing modality ground therapy promises to lower the cost of treatment for many diseases. And as the body of research confirming its benefits continues to grow, ground therapy units will likely become standard installations in spas, health clinics, and other health-centered locations such as hospitals and nursing homes. In other words, ground therapy holds the potential to generate a broad scientific and economic overhaul for the healthcare industry. For as Ober points out, ground therapy can improve not just our health, but also our economy.

As word spreads and the ground therapy revolution continues to gather speed, patients will begin to request to be grounded in hospitals and clinics around the world. Certainly, these requests may initially be ignored, or even ridiculed. But eventually, if the public continues to demand grounding in healthcare settings, hospitals and clinics will have to meet this demand. A hundred years from now, grounding as part of routine health care in hospitals and clinics will likely seem as obvious and undeniable a necessity as simple hand-washing and germ-control does today. It's important to remember that back when the germ theory was introduced, with its insistence on the need for basic sanitation in hospitals, it was severely ridiculed. As have been many of the world's most remarkable health advances.

Ultimately, as hospitals and clinics integrate grounding services, demand will grow for professionals who can work in ground therapy healthcare positions. Likewise, demand will grow for ground therapy products. Manufacturers will have to meet this demand by producing grounding mattresses, mats, and blankets.

The economic potential for a discovery like ground therapy is virtually unlimited. Not only do we stand to derive massive health benefits from this revolutionary healing modality, but we also stand to drastically cut health care costs and protecting our financial future. As our healthcare costs decline and come under control, the economic benefits from our increasing health and well-being, along with the growth of the ground therapy industry itself, will flourish and blossom.

The Road to Wellness

The road to wellness is often full obstacles, but they are obstacles worth overcoming. In the case of ground therapy, however, the obstacles are actually few once you make the initial decision to take the care of your health into your own hands. Once you do, you will see for yourself how little effort is required to gain massive health benefits. And in this sense, ground therapy is truly unique. We have grown accustomed to the idea that health-improving activities must be difficult, time consuming, and effortful. For instance, getting into great physical shape may involve a commitment to exercise, and eating well may require changing old habits that are so deeply ingrained that they seem impossible to break. But increasing our electron count is not difficult at all. In fact, it's so easy that you may not believe—at first—that it could possibly work. But it absolutely does!

When we are grounded, we are restored to the natural, holistic state nature intended. Our bodies know this, and they respond by regulating their physiological processes and healing damaged cells. Why would we *not* want to return to this state of peace and wellbeing? Ground therapy is fundamental for us as human beings, and it is crucial to maintaining our health.

Are *you* ready to get back in touch with your planet— and your health?

Chapter Eleven

Get Started With Ground Therapy

Each patient carries his own doctor inside him. They come to us now knowing this truth. We are at our best when they give the doctor who resides within each patient a chance to go to work. – Albert Schweitzer

Now that you have learned all about what grounding therapy can do for your health and wellbeing, you may be eager to try it. But you may be wondering how, exactly, you go about getting grounded. In this chapter you'll find everything you need to know about grounding so that you can get started right away. It's likely that you already have all the materials you need at hand, but before we get into the details of the method, there is one thing that you should keep in mind. The most conductive parts of your body are the soles of your feet and the palms of your hands, because there is always a little moisture in these locations, which facilitates electron transfer.

Grounding Yourself At Home

Walking or Running Barefoot

This is the easiest way to ground yourself, and it is just as effective as using a grounding tool such as a mat or conductivity rod. Simply take off your shoes and socks and walk on soft grass for a few minutes every day. It is best to do this on grass that is still slightly wet with dew, because wet grass is slightly more conductive. And try to do your barefoot walking in the first half of the day (before two o'clock in the afternoon), because the resulting stimulation of the nerves of the feet can cause problems with sleep if it occurs too close to bedtime.

Devices for Grounding

Some people require more time grounded than a barefoot walk can provide in order to experience the full benefits of ground therapy. Although you can make a grounding device at home (there are plenty of online tutorials that provide explanations and diagrams) most people simply prefer the convenience, safety, and appearance of manufactured grounding products over do-it-yourself devices. Conductive grounding devices are custom-designed and professionally manufactured, and are rigorously tested for effectiveness.

Grounding Recovery Bags

The first grounding recovery bag—called the Earthing Recovery Bag—was designed for Tour de France cyclists. This ground therapy option, which is like a typical sleeping bag except that it is made of conductive material, has become a popular sleeping accessory with athletes and travellers. According to grounding experts, many people also use grounding recovery bags in their own homes, "enjoying the effect of being cocooned in the earth's energy."

Grounding Beds

The Earthing Bed™ is currently the only grounding bed on the market. This specially designed Memory Foam mattress is made of organic cotton. What makes this mattress special, however, is that you simply need to plug it in to be connected to the earth's energy while you sleep. This is one of the most convenient ways to ground yourself, since it requires relatively little setup.

Conductive Grounding Sheets

Designed with the same technology as the Earthing Bed™, conductive grounding sheets are available from a handful of retailers. These sheets are typically all-natural, 100% cotton sheets made with a special conductive silver thread that grounds the sleeper to the earth. Typically, grounding sheets are fitted, allowing you to sleep on top of them. But you can also find half sheets, which go across the bottom of your bed, and which come into contact with your legs and feet only. Half sheets work just as well as the full ones, because as long as bare skin is in contact with the conductive sheet and it is plugged into the grounding hole of a grounding outlet, you receive the benefits of ground therapy. Grounding sheets are typically available in sizes to fit all standard beds.

Grounding Rods and Cords

If you are living in an older structure that does not have traditional outlets, you may be a candidate for a grounding rod. A grounding rod is composed of a conductive metal rod that can be stuck directly into the ground; attached to this rod is a cord that can be plugged into any grounding product. One tip from experts is that in arid climates or sandy soil, the ground rod should be watered weekly to improve conductivity. Even if the climate is not arid, watering the ground rod will help effectiveness whenever there has been no rain for a while.

Grounding Yourself at Work

You may think it would be more challenging to ground yourself at work than at home, since we often have less control over our work environment than we do of the environment in our homes. But grounding technology is equally convenient in our workplace thanks to a number of new grounding products.

Grounding Mats

Grounding mats offer a convenient and low-impact way to stay grounded in any environment. These mats are designed to be placed under your desk; the usual size is around 10 x 27 inches, which gives you ample space to rest your feet on them. If you opt for a grounding mat, look for one that is made of durable 100% natural rubber. The mats acquire their conductive ability from a matrix of highly conductive carbon particles hidden underneath the rubber cover.

Grounding Patches

Grounding patches are similar to the ECG/EKG electrode patches that medical professionals commonly use for testing purposes. To use the patches for grounding, they simply need to be attached to the body at a site of high conductivity (such as your palms or the soles of the feet) or a site of pain and sensitivity. The patches come with an accompanying grounding cord that attaches to the top of the patch and can be plugged into any wall outlet.

Grounding Yourself on the Go

Perhaps the hardest time to ground yourself is when you are traveling. When you are travelling it is sometimes difficult to find a wall outlet to plug in your grounding device. And when you are on the go you may not be in one place long enough to derive the full benefit from grounding. This is why grounding enthusiasts have now released a whole line of products designed specifically for those who wish to ground themselves on the go. Whether you are driving cross country, travelling halfway around the world, or simply out and about during the day doing your usual activities, these grounding products will allow you to benefit from being connected with the earth.

Grounding Outlet Adapters

If you are planning to travel outside of North America, keep in mind that the style and type of outlet may be different in your destination country, and may not fit products designed for North American use. In that case, you can purchase an adapter that will allow you to use your device in the United Kingdom, Australia, and Italy, as well as a universal (Type F) outlet adapter for Europe at large.

The Auto Seat Pad

Scientific evidence has recently confirmed that road vibration and related body motion on vehicle seats can generate micro-electrical charges in the body. Grounding pads for your car neutralize this charge, which means less strain and tension on a long driver, as Ober recently found in a study involving long-distance truck drivers. Auto seat pads are typically pads measuring 10" x 10" which are designed to be connected by a wire to the metal frame under the seat. If you are someone who drives long distances regularly, or are in your car frequently, an auto seat pad may be a great solution for you.

Grounding Shoes

Many ground therapy product manufacturers are now producing shoes that keep you grounded for the period of time that you are wearing them. For example, the designer Juil Hera has introduced a line of sandals for women called the Earthing Shoe. These sandals are leather-lined for maximum comfort, and they look almost identical to any other type of footwear, except for one detail: copper electrodes at the toes and heels to connect your feet to the earth. The Earthing Shoe gives you all the comfort of a leather interior and a polyurethane sole, but with the added health benefits of copper connectivity in the soles.

Grounding for Indoor Pets

Earlier we mentioned that animals are naturally shielded from EMF damage because they tend to be in constant (and unimpeded) contact with the earth. While this is true for animals living in a natural environment, it does not always hold for our family pets that live in the same insulated environments that we do, and often get little contact with the earth except for their daily walks. As a result, our beloved pets are becoming much more prone to developing health problems similar to those that pose a threat for us.

And according to Dr. Stephen Blake, a homeopathic veterinarian San Diego, pets can benefit equally as well as their owners do from grounding. In fact, grounding pads especially designed for pets are now available. These pads, which are small enough to fit on doggie or cat beds, are padded for maximum comfort. And like any other grounding product, they plug directly into any wall outlet.

Dr. Blake describes the astonishing results that one of his patients, Jackson, experienced from sleeping on a grounding pad. Jackson, a 16-year-old blind lap dog, was suffering from many ailments, including arthritis and fatigue. But as Dr. Blake observed, sleeping grounded resulted in a marked improvement in his symptoms and discomfort level. So much so, in fact, that Jackson began to protest when his grounding pad was removed from his bed for laundering!

> *Jackson is a 16-year-old blind pup who has a fit when his caregiver takes his [grounding pad] up to wash the cover . . . He is feeling much better since he can now ground himself and help his body absorb the negative electrons it needs to stay in balance.* – Dr. Stephen Blake

Clint Ober has also observed the way in which grounding can help relieve the suffering of animals—and speed healing after injury. As a young child, Ober remembers seeing an injured calf lying on the ground at his family farm. The calf had sustained a very extensive wound to its stomach, possibly from a wild animal attack, and was bleeding profusely. Ober's father attempted to help the calf by sewing up the wound with a needle and coarse thread, but with no antiseptics or antibiotics on hand, it seemed obvious to everyone in attendance that the calf's chances of survival were dismal. To add to the risk, they were miles from the barn, with no way to get the calf safely to shelter. They had no other choice but to leave the injured calf lying on the ground where it had fallen, guarded protectively by its mother. Within a week, that little calf was running around the farm, cavorting with the other calves as if nothing had happened. Ober realized that the only way that the calf could be so fully healed from this traumatic injury—let alone healed so quickly—was through its connection to the earth. Lying on the ground with its whole body pressed to the ground had allowed electrons to flood the calf's body, restoring homeostasis and hastening the healing process.

The only conclusion we can draw from stories like this is when even our pets benefit from being grounded, we know that we have a truly revolutionary medical technology on our hands.

The Road to Wellness

As we have stressed throughout this book, ground therapy is such a wonderful health practice not only because it is so *effective*, but also because it can be done on a small budget—or even for free—so it is a healing modality that is truly available to everyone. And it's possibly the most convenient form of health care ever, because you can do it while sleeping, working, playing with the kids, walking the dog, and even while you're cooking! And thanks to the line of professionally designed products now available, we can derive all the benefits of standing barefoot outside virtually anywhere. And as more and more research confirms the true power of grounding, we believe that we will discover that it is a healing option that virtually has no limits!

Don't we all owe it to ourselves to reconnect with the earth and live long, healthy, and vibrant lives?

Epilogue

Ground Therapy for Your Future

To keep the body in good health is a duty—otherwise we shall not be able to keep our mind strong and clear.

– Buddha

G round therapy not only offers you better health right now—it also contributes to a longer and far healthier future. Stabilizing your body with the earth's electrons is a proven way to raise your chances of greater longevity and an improved quality of life. In other words, ground therapy offers you the very real opportunity to age gracefully and in optimum health, without the typical age-related issues such as disease, limited mobility, and fatigue. In other words, choosing to practice grounding is actually a way of making an investment in your own future.

And if we don't make this investment, a terrifying future may loom. The fact that the youngest generation in America is expected to have a shorter average lifespan than their parents is not only shocking, but it also highlights a very frightening possibility. And if this trend continues unchecked, humankind may well eventually become an endangered species!

However, it should be stressed—and stressed again!— that this need not be our eventuality. Ground therapy is a healing modality like no other, because it has not only the potential to heal our current health woes, but also to reverse the outcomes of the downward health spiral that we now face for the future.

And there is one other benefit of ground therapy that has yet to be mentioned, but that is inextricably linked with the health of the world's peoples. The connection we reestablish with the earth through grounding is almost spiritual in nature. We are reminded of how we were meant to live, and how we were meant to feel before the stressors of modern life caused our bodies to go haywire. And by reawakening to this awareness of our intrinsic connection to the earth, many people find that they also become inspired to live in a more natural, organic way. And this is not only good news for us and the people we love—it is also very good for the earth which supports, nurtures, and heals us as well.

Earthing is the future. Humanity needs to reconnect to the planet, to our natural electrical state, and to our natural state of good health...Wake up, people. Go out. Ground yourself. Reintroduce your bare feet to the ground. Sleep grounded, and, if you can, work grounded, play grounded, and watch TV grounded. If you haven't done it by now, go sit or stand barefoot outside (weather permitting) for a half hour or so. If you have pain, see what difference it makes. Then ask yourself if reconnecting with the Earth might be the most amazing health discovery you have ever made. – Clint Ober

Index

birth defects 10

bladder 87, 90

Blake, Dr. Stephen 149

blood cells 47, 50, 51, 54-55, 102, 105

  agglutination (clumping) 54

  red blood cell clumping (RBC) 104

  white 47

blood clotting 48, 76

blood flow 3, 76, 99

blood pressure 11, 74, 101, 115

blood sugar (see glucose)

blood viscosity 97, 102-104, 115

body electric, the 6

Body Electric, The (Robert Becker) 7

bowel habits, changes in 90

bradycardia 100

brain, the 7, 10, 20, 36, 113-114

  tumors of 10

brainwaves 53

breasts, lumps or thickening in 91

breath, shortness of 100

Briffa, Dr. John 52

Buddha 153

C

California Institute for Human Science, The 61

carbohydrates 121

carbon dioxide 91

cancer 3, 9, 10, 24, 29, 34, 37, 71, 75-77, 85-93, 95, 98-99, 109, 123-126, 135

  causes of 88-91

  predicted death rates (2013) by type of 87

  symptoms of 90-91

carcinogens 9, 88

cardiovascular disease 45, 100, 102-103, 104, 105, 115

  symptoms of 100

Carnegie Mellon University 70

carpal tunnel syndrome 52, 92, 133

cataracts 10

celiac disease 35

cells, damage to 47-48, 88-89, 92, 123, 141

  inter-communication between 74, 113, 117, 131

Centers for Disease Control and Prevention, The (CDC) 64, 108, 109

chakra 5

chee gong (qi gong) 5

chemical reactions 8, 39

chemotherapy 138

Chevalier, Gáetan 59-61, 65-67, 103

Chinese Medicine (See Traditional Chinese Medicine)

chronic inflammation (see inflammation, chronic)

chronic obstructive pulmonary disease (COPD) 126

cigarette smoke 88, 125

circadian rhythms (also see sleep) 23, 80, 82

circulation (see blood flow)

cirrhosis of the liver 126

cognitive imbalance 1

congestive heart failure 24

constipation 52, 133

coronary bypass surgery 138

cortisol (epinephrine) 18, 69, 72, 78-82, 93

circadian cortisol test 80

cough 91

cystic fibrosis 126

Czeisler, Dr. Charles 110-111

160

√ If you enjoyed this book ...
and you wish to order more copies
to give away to friends and family members, go to

http://www.GroundTherapy.com

√ Discover other health secrets and
little-known health discoveries by subscribing to
the *Underground Health Reporter*™ e-newsletter
for FREE at:

http://www.UndergroundHealthReporter.com

√ To see our other book titles, go to:

http://www.ThinkOutsideTheBook.com

or contact
Think-Outside-the-Book Publishing, LLC
311 N. Robertson Boulevard, Suite 323
Beverly Hills, California 90211

info@ThinkOutsideTheBook.com

(323) 331-9316